Ketogenic Diet

Appetizers and Condiments Cookbook

How to Lose Weight Quickly, Turn Fat into Energy and Prevent Disease to Live Healthily

Amelia Ramos

Table of Contents

Introduction

You can not

think well, love well, sleep well,

if you haven't eaten well.

Virginia Woolf

A ketogenic diet, which requires a low carb, moderate protein and high fat nutritional intake has become increasingly popular in recent years as more and more people are looking for a nutritional approach to optimize their health.

Let's see together the recipes that belong to this diet.

Small poetic license:

in the book I often used "cup" as a unit of measurement; this to give even more simplicity to the Keto world, which does not need sling bars, perfect grams etc., but is a very, very simple way of doing it within everyone's reach.

I hope I enjoyed it.

Appetizers

Herb Salmon Sauce

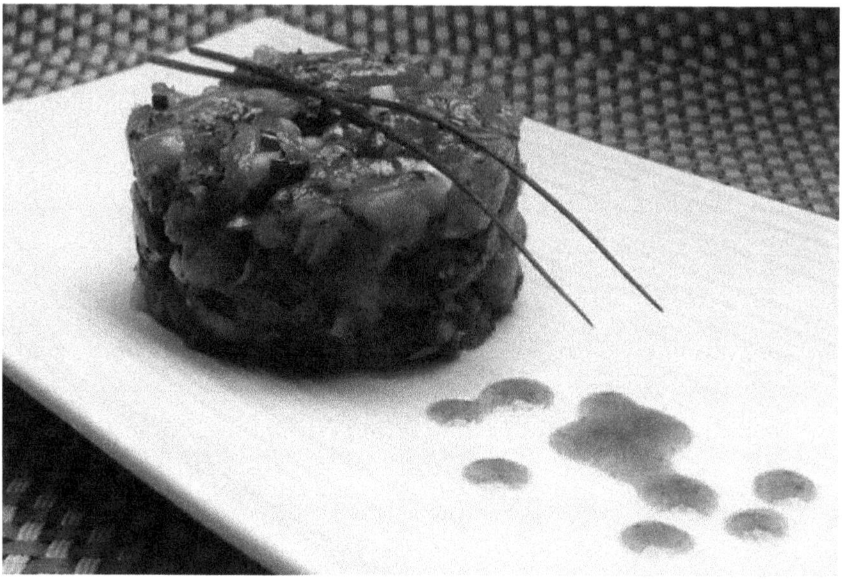

KETO - WITHOUT NUTS

Preparation time: 5 minutes, plus 1 hour to chill

Yield: 8 servings

My mom always serves it at family gatherings, and it's one of my favorite dishes. I love it with celery, pickles, fried keto bread.

170 grams of cream cheese, softened

3 tablespoons of mayonnaise

1 tablespoon of lime juice

½ teaspoon of fine sea salt

2 teaspoons of chopped fresh dill

⅛ teaspoon of freshly ground black pepper

1 homemade salmon recipe

2 green onions, thinly sliced

1. In a medium-sized bowl, combine the cream cheese, mayonnaise, lime juice, salt, dill, and pepper; mix until well combined and smooth. Gently stir in the salmon and green onions.

2. Cover and refrigerate for at least 1 hour. Store in an airtight container in the refrigerator for up to 5 days.

Nutritional information (per serving)

145 calories

fat 12.8 g 79%

proteins 6.9 g 19%

carbohydrates 1 g 3%

fiber 0 g

Tray of appetizers

KETO - WITHOUT NUTS

Preparation time: 2 minutes

Yield: 6 servings

Arrange the cheese slices on a large platter or cutting board. Drizzle with olive oil and sprinkle with fresh herbs and a pinch of salt and pepper. Add the olives and meat to the tray and serve.

350 grams of fresh mozzarella, cut into rounds

2 tablespoons of high quality extra virgin olive oil or MCT oil

2 tablespoons of chopped fresh basil and / or oregano

Fine sea salt and freshly ground black pepper

24 pitted olives of your choice

100 grams of salami, thinly sliced

Nutritional information (per serving)

calories 289

fats 21.9 g 68%

protein 18.8 g 26%

carbohydrates 4.1 g 6%

fibers 0.9 g

Beef carpaccio

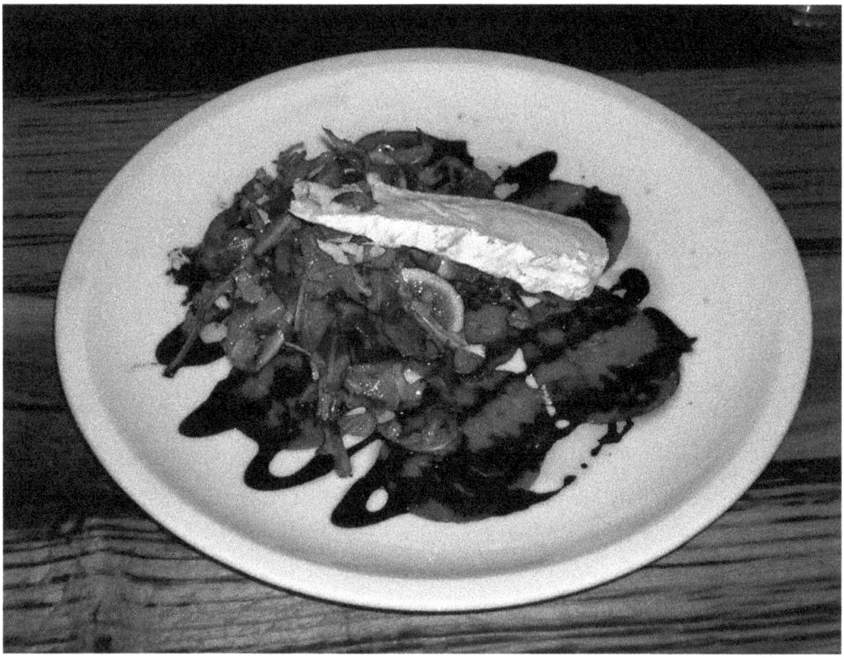

KETO - WITHOUT NUTS

Preparation time: 10 minutes, plus 2 hours to cool the fillet

Yield: 4 servings

200 grams of thinly sliced beef fillet or bresaola

4 tablespoons of fat-burning salad dressing

2 cups of rocket

½ cup diced yellow tomatoes

¼ cup of capers

50 grams of Parmesan, freshly chopped (about ½ cup)

½ teaspoon of fine sea salt

½ teaspoon of freshly ground black pepper

1. If using the fillet: wrap the fillet in parchment paper and place it in the freezer for 2 hours. Once semi-frozen, unwrap and slice the beef into thin pieces. Arrange the slices on a sheet of parchment paper. Top with another piece of parchment and lightly pound the meat with a meat mallet until thin. Repeat until all the beef slices are pounded thin.

2. Arrange the slices of fillet or bresaola on a serving dish, overlapping them slightly. Pour all but 1 1/2 teaspoons of salad dressing over the meat.

3. Mix the arugula, tomatoes and capers with the remaining salad dressing and arrange over the meat. Sprinkle with the Parmesan, salt and pepper.

Busy family tip: You can save time by asking your butcher to pound the meat for you.

Note: If you don't want to use raw beef for this recipe, use bresaola, which is cured red meat.

Nutritional information (per serving)

256 calories

fat 17,8 g 63%

proteins 21.7 g 34%

carbohydrates 1.9 g 3%

fibers 0,6 g

Endive stuffed with chicken curry

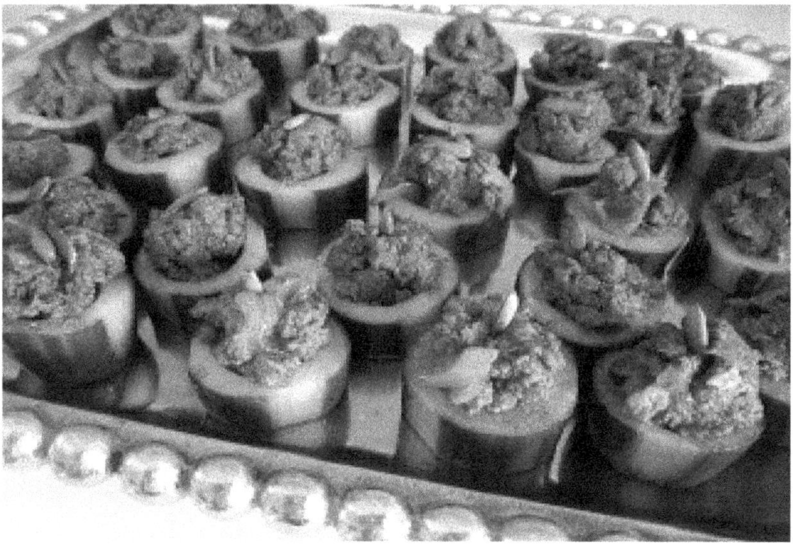

KETO - NO NUTS - NO LACTOSE

Preparation time: 15 minutes, plus 3 hours to chill

Cooking time: 1 hour and 45 minutes

Yield: 12 servings

3 tablespoons of MCT oil, bacon fat or lard

1 kg of chicken thigh quarters

2 teaspoons of fine sea salt, divided

1 teaspoon of freshly ground black pepper

¼ cup diced yellow onion

1 head of roasted garlic

2 cups of chicken bone broth

1 cup diced celery

¼ cup chopped green onions, white and green parts

1 1/2 cups of mayonnaise

1/4 cup chopped dill pickles

3 tablespoons of curry powder

3 heads of white and / or red endive, without leaves and cleaned

Sliced or diced red onion, for garnish (optional)

Necessary material

KITCHEN ROBOT

1. Heat the MCT oil in a deep skillet over medium-high heat. Season the chicken with 1 teaspoon of salt and pepper. Place the chicken in the hot oil and brown it for about 8 minutes, or until golden on all sides.

2. Add the diced onion to the pot and squeeze the roasted garlic from the head into the pot. Cook over medium heat for about 8 minutes, stirring occasionally, until the onion is golden.

3. Add the broth, reduce the heat and simmer, covered, for about 1 1/2 hours, until the chicken is almost detached from the bone. Remove the chicken from the pan and let it cool slightly so you can handle it.

4. Remove the meat from the bones and cut into small pieces, retaining the bones and the liquid to make the bone broth. Place the chicken pieces, celery and green onions in a mixing bowl.

5. In the bowl of a food processor, combine the mayonnaise, dill pickles, curry powder, and the remaining 1 teaspoon of salt. Blend until smooth.

6. Pour the dressing over the chicken and vegetables and mix to coat evenly. Refrigerate for a few hours to let the flavors blend.

7. Serve at room temperature in endive leaves, about 2 tablespoons per leaf. Garnish with red onion if desired.

Nutritional information (per serving)

378 calories

fat 32,8 g 78%

protein 15.3 g 16%

carbohydrates 7.2 g 8%

fibers 4.9 g

Grilled Halloumi - with ham and pesto

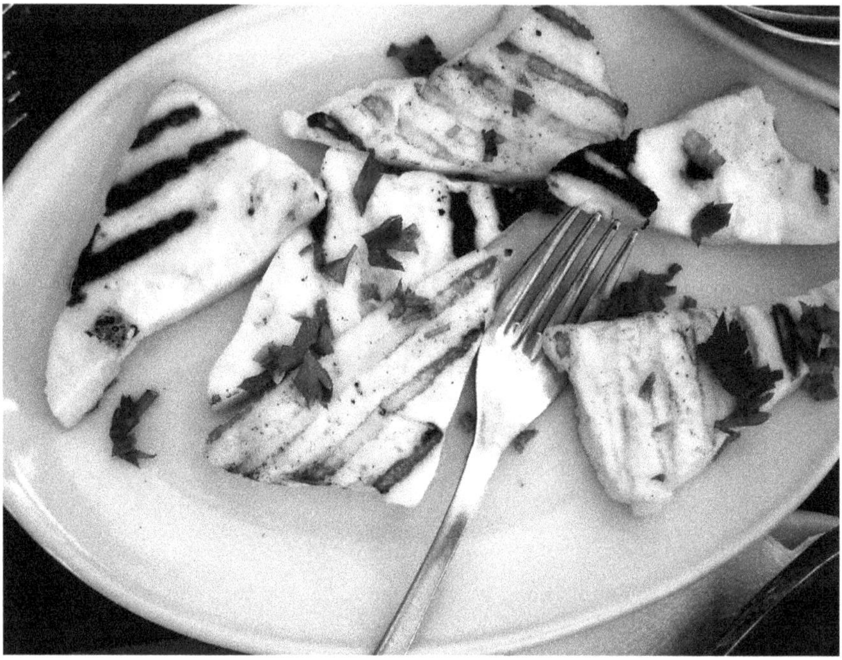

KETO - NO NUTS - NO LACTOSE

Preparation time: 5 minutes

Cooking time: 12 minutes

Yield: 6 servings

Halloumi is a slightly chewy and compact cheese, delicious but on the salty side. The texture reminds me of a thick feta, but has a different flavor profile. Halloumi has a unique quality: you can grill it or fry it! When heated, Halloumi becomes creamy and its salinity fades, turning it into a robust and flavorful bite.

200 grams of Halloumi cheese, cut into slices

1 tablespoon MCT oil or melted unsalted butter

6 slices of ham

¼ cup of pesto

1/2 cup chopped yellow tomato

Fresh marjoram or basil leaves, for garnish (optional)

1. Preheat a grill or sandwich maker over medium-high heat.

2. Brush each side of the cheese slices with MCT oil or melted butter. Place on hot grill or sandwich maker for 3 minutes on each side, or until golden brown with grill marks. Meanwhile, arrange the ham on a serving plate, leaving some space between each slice.

3. Remove the cheese slices from the grill and divide them equally between the ham. Sprinkle evenly with the pesto and yellow tomato. Sprinkle some fresh marjoram or basil leaves around the dish if desired. Serve hot.

Nutritional information (per serving)

calories 185

fat 15 g 73%

protein 11.3 g 24%

carbohydrates 1.3 g 3%

fibers 0 g

Pan-fried ham - stretched curd cheeses

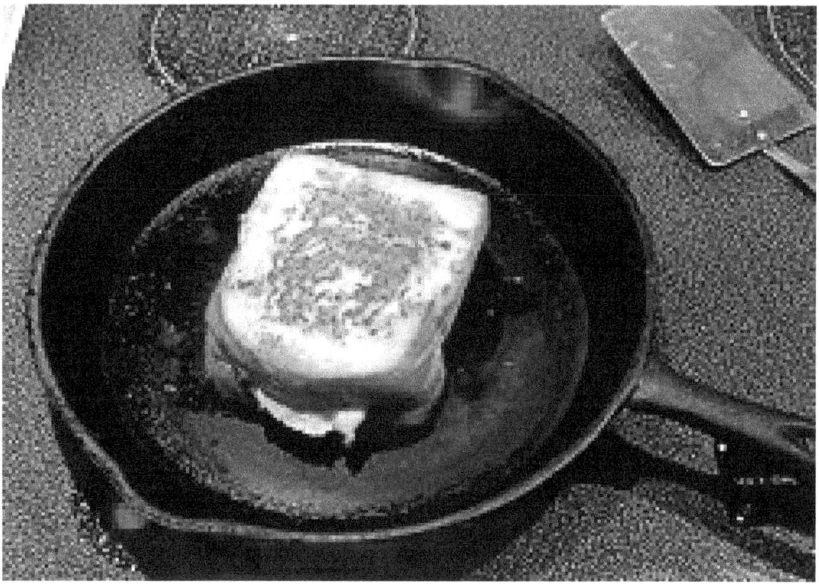

KETO - WITHOUT NUTS

Preparation time: 10 minutes

Cooking time: 4 minutes

Yield: 8 pieces (2 per serving)

2 tablespoons of MCT oil

2 tablespoons of unsalted butter

8 pieces of stretched curd cheese, frozen

8 very thin slices of ham

Fresh chopped herbs, such as sage, tarragon, or thyme (optional)

Marinara sauce, homemade or store bought, by dipping (optional)

1. Heat the MCT oil and butter in a sauté pan over medium-high heat. Discard the cheese.

2. Wrap a piece of ham around each piece of string cheese, making sure to cover all the cheese and the edges. The ham will stick to the cheese. If desired, roll the ham-coated cheese in chopped herbs for a crunchy herb crust.

3. Place each stick of cheese wrapped in frozen ham in the hot oil and fry, turning often, until the outside is slightly crisp and the cheese is sticky. It will only take a few minutes.

4. Remove on a serving dish, allow to cool slightly and enjoy with marinara sauce!

Nutritional information (per serving)

334 calories

fat 28.4 g 76%

protein 17,3 g 21%

carbohydrates 2 g 3%

fibers 0 g

Celery boats

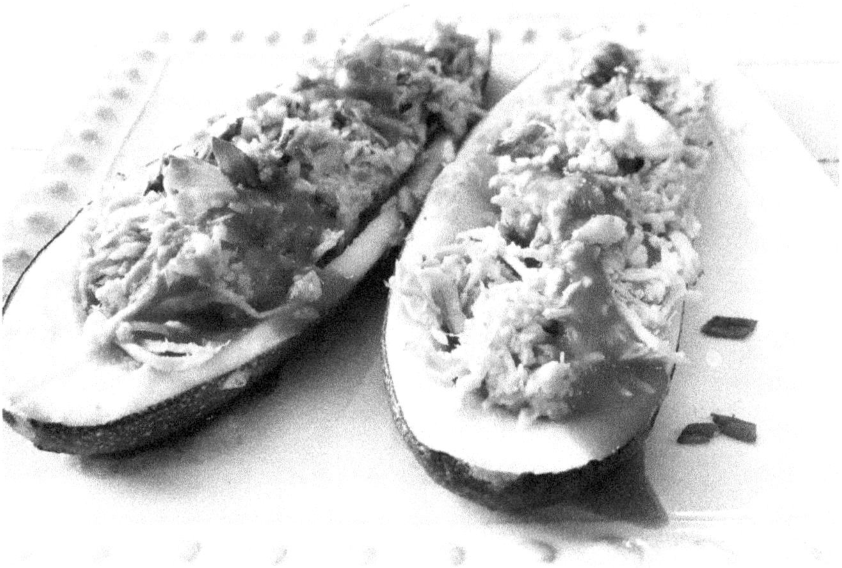

KETO - NO NUTS - NO LACTOSE

Preparation time: 15 minutes

Cooking time: 12 minutes

Yield: 8 servings (2 boats per serving)

I garnished this dish with hibiscus sea salt, which is typically used in Spanish cooking and adds a nice purple color. But if you can't find hibiscus salt, you can also season it with regular sea salt.

4 large eggs

¼ cup of mayonnaise

1 tablespoon of Dijon mustard

1 1/2 teaspoons chopped fresh dill or your favorite herb

1 teaspoon of paprika

Fine sea salt and freshly ground black pepper to taste

8 large stalks of celery

16 pitted black olives

Fresh dill, for garnish

1. Place the eggs in a saucepan and cover with cold water. Bring the water to a boil, cover and remove from the heat. Let the eggs sit in the hot water for 10-12 minutes. Remove the eggs from the hot water, place them in a bowl of ice water to cool and peel. Cut the eggs into ¼-inch slices.

2. Burst the yolks of 16 slices and reserve the egg whites to make the sails. In a large bowl, combine the rest of the egg slices and egg yolks, mayonnaise, mustard, dill, paprika, salt and pepper. Mash well with a fork or wooden spoon.

3. Using a peeler, cut a thin slice along the rounded side of each celery stick so that the celery sticks can be open side up without wobbling. Cut the celery sticks into sixteen 7cm long pieces and fill them with the egg salad.

4. Place an olive inside each reserved egg white slice. Place a toothpick on one side of the egg white, the olive and the other side of the egg white, so that it retains its shape.

5. Stick the toothpick with the egg white sail into the edge of a celery boat. Garnish with sea salt and dill.

Nutritional information (per serving)

192 calories
fats 17,2 g 81%
protein 7 g 15%

carbohydrates 3.2 g 7%
fibers 1,5 g

Ham salad

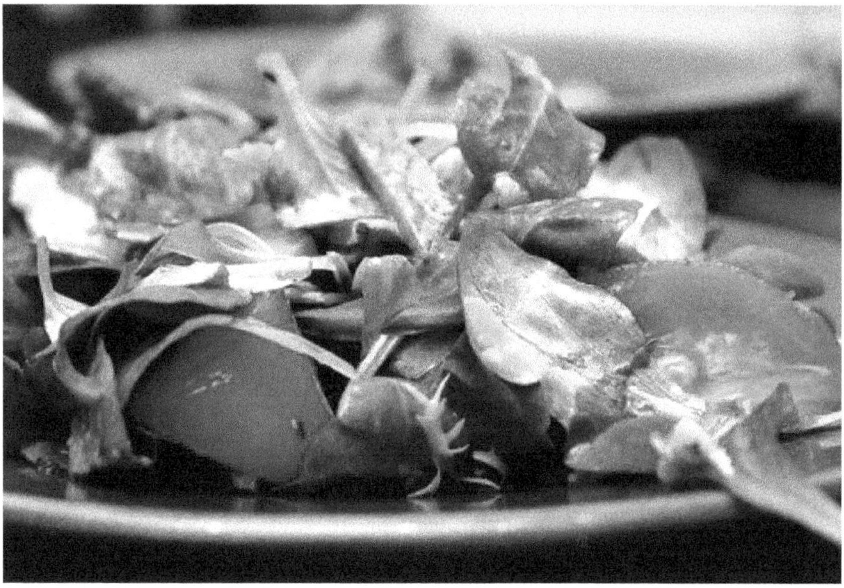

KETO - NO NUTS - NO LACTOSE

Preparation time: 15 minutes

Cooking time: 12 minutes

Yield: 12 servings

2 large eggs

3 cups of fully ground cooked ham

2 tablespoons of finely chopped celery

1 tablespoon plus 1 teaspoon finely diced dill pickles, plus more for garnish (optional)

2 teaspoons diced green onions

1 cup of mayonnaise

1 tablespoon of your favorite homemade mustard

⅓ small cucumber, for serving

1 tablespoon diced red onion, for garnish (optional)

1. Place the eggs in a saucepan and cover with cold water. Bring the water to a boil, cover and remove from the heat. Let the eggs sit in the hot water for 10-12 minutes. Remove the eggs from the hot water and place them in a bowl of ice water to cool. Peel and chop the eggs.

2. In a large bowl, combine the chopped eggs, ham, celery, pickles, and green onions. Combine the mayonnaise and mustard in a separate bowl, then pour the ham mixture over it. Stir to coat. Refrigerate until ready to serve.

3. To serve, cut the cucumber into slices. Place 1 1/2 tablespoons of ham salad on each cucumber slice. Garnish with diced pickles and red onion if desired.

Nutritional information (per serving)

calories 189

fats 17.1 g 81%

protein 6.7 g 14%

carbohydrates 1,8 g 4%

fibers 0.5 g

Mini-frico

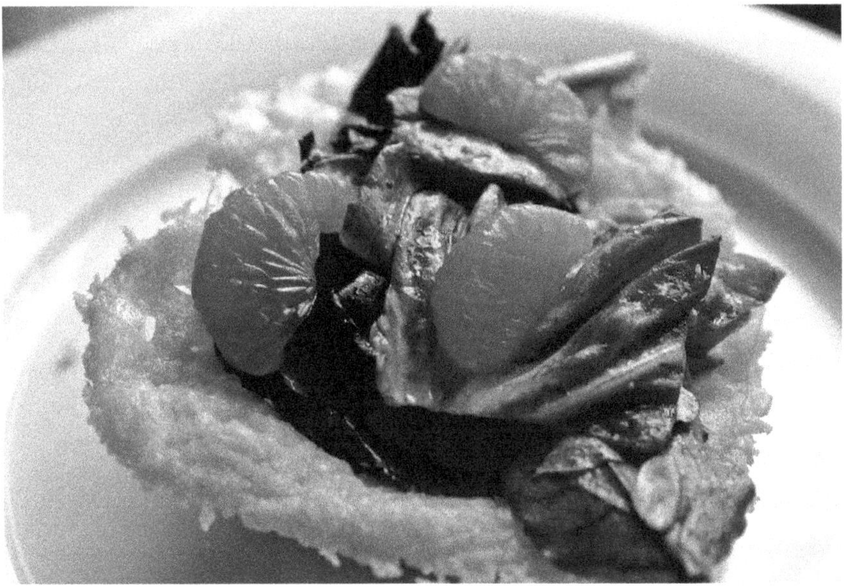

KETO - WITHOUT NUTS

Preparation time: 15 minutes

Cooking time: 10 minutes

Yield: 12 cups of frico (1 per serving)

Frico is an Italian dish that basically consists of crispy fried cheese. What's not to love about this? Making these appetizers may seem daunting at first, but once you get the hang of it, they're very simple to make. Make sure you have the filling ready to serve just before serving; if you fill the frico cups too early before serving, they can become a little soft and lose their crunchiness.

2 cups grated Parmesan (about 8 ounces)

For the filling

1 cup of chopped arugula

4 slices of bacon, cooked and crumbled into small pieces

1 cup quartered yellow tomatoes

2 tablespoons of mayonnaise

1/4 cup roughly chopped fresh flat-leaf parsley

60 grams of cheese, crumbled (about ½ cup), for garnish

1. Preheat the oven to 190 ° C. Line a baking sheet lined with parchment paper.

2. Place 1 large tablespoon of Parmesan in a 6cm jar or cookie cutter and use your fingers to spread the cheese to fill the lid, forming a circle. Then flip the cheese over the prepared baking sheet. Repeat until you have 6 circles of cheese, keeping them about 5 centimeters apart on the pan.

3. Cook the cheese rolls for 5 minutes or until lightly golden and bubbly. Once out of the oven, they start to harden, so you need to work quickly. Use a spatula or knife to transfer the rounds to a muffin pan and press gently to form a cup. If the rolls get too cold and brittle to shape, put them back in the hot oven for 30 seconds so they become flexible again.

4. Allow the cheese cups to cool in the mini muffin pan for 5 minutes and remove. Repeat the entire process with the rest of the cheese, for a total of 12 cups.

5. Put the rocket, bacon, yellow tomatoes and mayonnaise in a small bowl and mix well to combine. Fill each cup of frico with 2 tablespoons of the rocket mixture. Garnish with the parsley and gorgonzola and serve.

Nutritional information (per serving)

calories 131
fat 10.1 g 69%

protein 9.1 g 28%
carbohydrates 1,4 g 4%
fibers 0 g

Blt Bites

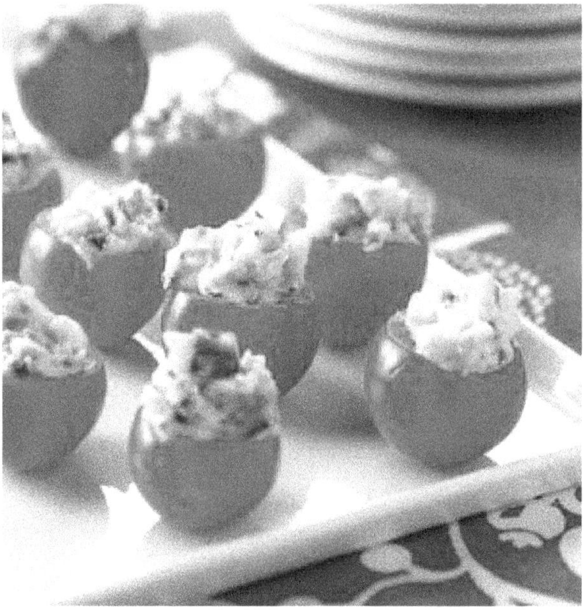

KETO - NO NUTS - NO LACTOSE

Preparation time: 10 minutes

Cooking time: 30 minutes

Yield: 16 bites (2 per serving)

2 tablespoons of coconut oil, to grease the pan

12 slices of bacon

1 cup of rocket

6 tablespoons homemade ranch dressing, regular or dairy-free or mayonnaise, plus more for garnish (optional)

¼ cup of chopped cherry tomatoes

2 tablespoons of chopped chives

1. Preheat the oven to 190 ° C. Turn a muffin pan over and place it on a rimmed baking sheet (to catch the fat). Grease the bottom of the muffin pan turned upside down, which is facing up.

2. Cut 8 slices of bacon in half crosswise, making 16 half sections. Cut the other 4 slices crosswise into 4 even sections each, making 16 smaller quarters. To make 1 cup of bacon, you will need 1 quarter of bacon and 1 half section of bacon.

3. Place one of the quarter pieces of bacon on top of an inverted muffin cup. Take one of the longer slices and wrap it around the sides of the muffin cup, overlapping it as much as possible between the 2 pieces because the bacon will shrink. Secure the ends with a toothpick. Repeat until you have set 16 cups of bacon.

4. Bake for 27-30 minutes or until golden but not overly crunchy (if they are too crunchy, it will be impossible to remove them from the pan). Remove from the oven and let cool for a few minutes, then gently remove from the pan. Let it cool completely.

5. Meanwhile, chop the rocket and stir in the ranch dressing. Once cooled, fill each cup with the seasoned rocket, a few pieces of chopped cherry tomatoes and a sprinkling of chives. If desired, add extra dressing on top.

Nutritional information (per serving)

calories 274

fat 25 g 82%

proteins 10 g 14%

carbohydrates 3 g 4%

fibers 0 g

Meatballs nirvana

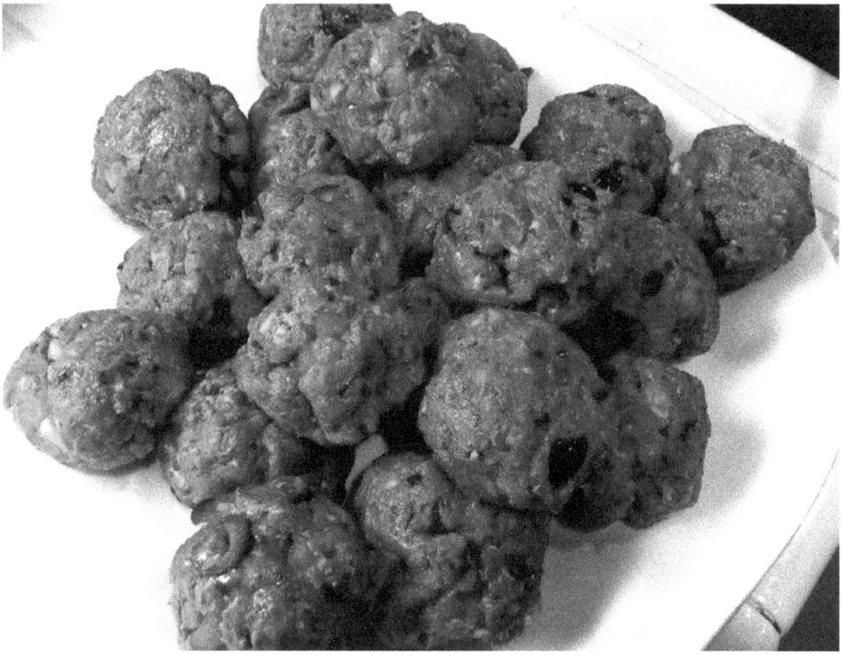

KETO - WITHOUT NUTS

Preparation time: 8 minutes

Cooking time: 15 minutes

Yield: 8 servings

200 grams of ground pork

200 grams of ground chicken (preferably dark meat)

60 grams of cream cheese (about ¼ cup), softened

2 large eggs

2 tablespoons of finely chopped celery

1 to 3 tablespoons of crumbled cheese, depending on taste

1 teaspoon of fine sea salt

½ teaspoon of freshly ground black pepper

For the sauce

½ cup unsalted melted butter or coconut oil

1/2 cup hot sauce of your choice, such as buffalo wing sauce

To serve

½ cup of homemade ranch dressing, regular or dairy-free

Celery stalks

Pieces of blue cheese

1. Preheat the oven to 180 ° C. Line a baking sheet lined with baking paper.

2. In a medium bowl, combine the ground pork, ground chicken, cream cheese, eggs, celery, blue cheese, salt, and pepper. The mixture will be sticky. Shape into 2.5 cm balls.

3. Place the meatballs on the prepared baking sheet and cook for 15 minutes. Once the meatballs are cooked, take them out of the oven and place them in a serving bowl.

4. Combine the butter and hot sauce in a small bowl. Pour the sauce over the meatballs and mix gently to coat.

5. Serve with the ranch dressing, celery sticks and blue cheese.

Tip: Before making balls, test the sauce by making a small pie and baking it. The mixture should taste amazing! If it doesn't, it probably needs more salt.

Nutritional information (per serving)

calories 282

fats 22.3 g 71%

protein 19.2 g 27%

carbohydrates 1 g 1%

fibers 0 g

Greek meze

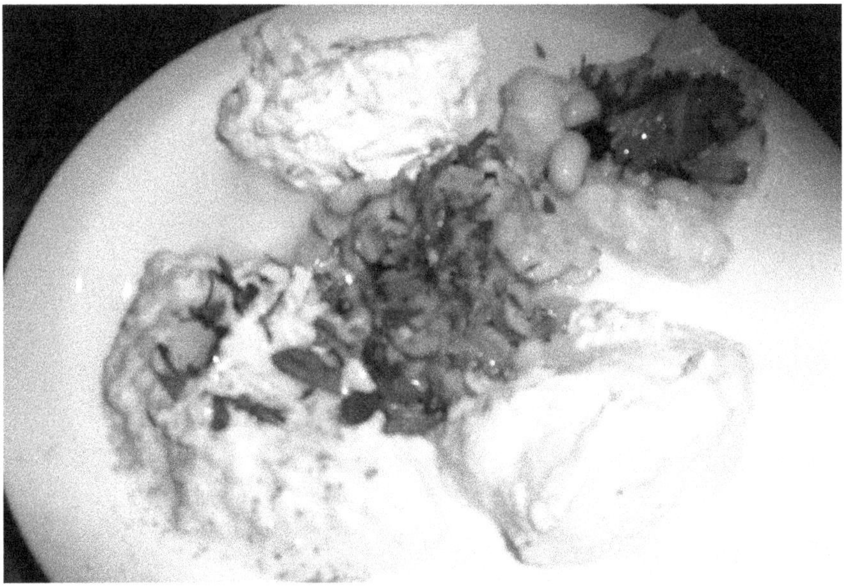

KETO - WITHOUT NUTS

Preparation time: 8 minutes

Yield: 16 meze bites (2 per person)

1 cucumber, cut into thick slices

¼ teaspoon of fine sea salt

¼ teaspoon of freshly ground black pepper

4 slices of salami, cut into quarters

100 grams of feta cheese, cut into 16 small cubes

8 cherry tomatoes or cherry tomatoes, cut in half

16 pitted olives

2 tablespoons of Greek salad dressing

1. Place the cucumber slices on a large serving dish and season with salt and pepper. Place a quarter of salami on top of the cucumber, then add a cube of feta, a tomato half and an olive. Insert a toothpick into the stack to secure it.

2. Season with the dressing and serve.

Nutritional information (per serving)

120 calories

fats 8.3 g 62%

protein 4.9 g 16%

carbohydrates 7.1 g 23%

fibers 1.6 g

Spring rolls

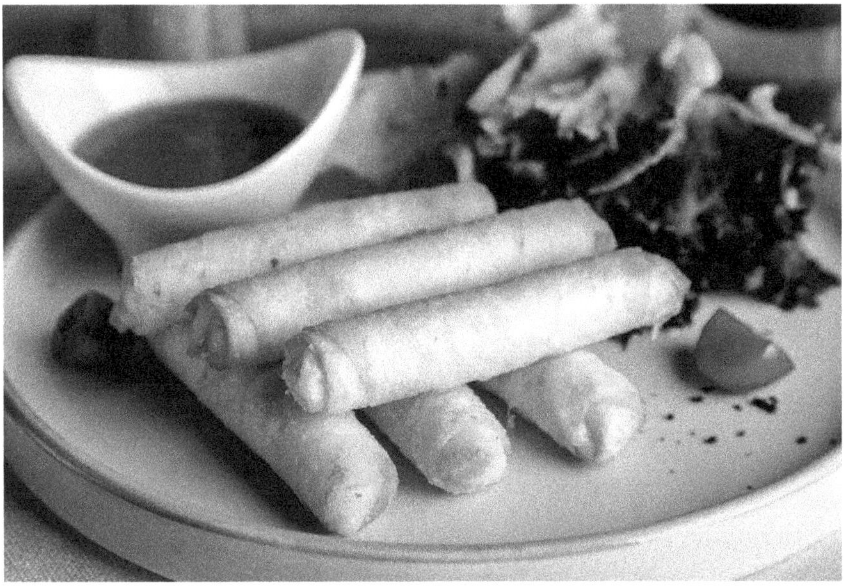

KETO - NO NUTS - NO LACTOSE

Preparation time: 15 minutes, plus 10 minutes to marinate the filling

Cooking time: 10 minutes

Yield: 8 spring rolls (2 per serving)

For the bands

3 liters of water

1 tablespoon of fine sea salt

1 head of green or purple cabbage

Coriander, scallion, or chives stalks to tie the rolls (optional)

For the filling

200 grams of ground pork or chicken

1/4 cup finely chopped green onions

2 tablespoons of fresh flat-leaf parsley cut

2 cloves of garlic, minced

1 tablespoon of MCT oil or dark sesame oil

2 teaspoons of lime juice

1 teaspoon of fresh grated ginger

½ teaspoon of fine sea salt

¼ teaspoon of grated lime zest

¼ teaspoon of freshly ground black pepper

1 tablespoon of coconut oil, for frying

For the dipping sauce

¼ cup of beef bone broth

3 tablespoons coconut oil (no substitutes, it will thicken the cooled sauce)

2 tablespoons of lime juice

2 tablespoons of powdered erythritol or 1 drop of stevia glycerite

1 tablespoon of almond butter

1 tablespoon of coconut aminos or grain-free tamari sauce

1 teaspoon of fish sauce

1 teaspoon of fresh grated ginger

½ clove of minced garlic

1. Prepare the rolls: Fill a 4 to 5-quart saucepan with 3 liters of water and 1 tablespoon of salt and bring to a boil.

2. Meanwhile, take an ice water bath in a large bowl.

3. Remove the 8 outer leaves from the cabbage. Make a cut through each individual leaf at the base where it attaches to the core. Cut off part of the woody area of the stem from the leaf. Set the rest of the head of cabbage aside to use for the filling.

4. Put the 8 cabbage leaves in boiling water; blanch for 30 seconds to 1 minute, until wilted. Quickly cool by soaking the cabbage leaves in ice water for 1 minute. Remove the leaves from the water and lay them on a cloth to dry.

5. Prepare the filling: Finely chop about 2 cups of cabbage from the rest of the head.

6. In a large bowl, combine the chopped cabbage with the stuffing ingredients (except coconut oil) and marinate for at least 10 minutes (or overnight) in the refrigerator.

7. Heat a large skillet over high heat. When hot, stir in a spoonful of coconut oil. Stir-fry the ground pork filling until golden brown. Transfer the browned filling to a bowl and set aside.

8. Assemble the rolls: take a blanched cabbage leaf and lay it flat, with the end of the base towards you. Place ¼ cup of the filling in the center of the leaf. Fold the end of the base over the filling and fold both sides in and over the filling so that it closes the open edges. Continue rolling to the end of the leaf, wrapping it tightly. Tie with a stalk of cilantro, green onion, or chives, if desired. Repeat with the remaining leaves and the filling.

9. Make the dipping sauce: In a small saucepan, combine all the sauce ingredients and heat over medium heat, whisking constantly, until very smooth. Remove the sauce from the heat, pour it into a serving dish and let it cool completely before serving.

Note: Homemade bone broth creates a thicker sauce. Broth or store-bought beef broth will work, but the sauce won't be as thick.

Nutritional information (per serving)

calories 288

fats 22 g 69%

protein 19 g 26%

carbohydrates 3.5 g 5%

fibers 0,6 g

Cheese curd wrapped in bacon

KETO - WITHOUT NUTS

Preparation time: 10 minutes

Cooking time: 8 minutes

Yield: 4 servings

2 tablespoons of MCT oil

2 tablespoons of unsalted butter

60 grams of bacon

100 grams of cheese curd, frozen

2 tablespoons chopped fresh herbs, such as cilantro or flat-leaf parsley (optional)

¼ cup barbecue mustard or ketchup keto, for serving

1. Heat the MCT oil and butter in a sauté pan over medium-high heat.

2. Wrap a piece of bacon around each frozen cheese curd, taking care to completely cover the cheese. Secure the bacon with a toothpick. If desired, roll bacon-wrapped cheese curd in chopped herbs for a crispy herb crust.

3. Working in batches to avoid overcrowding the pan, place the cheese curd wrapped in hot oil, turning it often, until the outside is slightly crunchy and the cheese becomes sticky. This will only take a few minutes per batch.

4. Transfer to a serving dish, allow to cool slightly and enjoy with mustard or ketchup.

Busy Families Tip: You can freeze bacon-wrapped cheese curd until you're ready to fry it.

Variation: cheese wrapped in ham. Replace the bacon with 60 grams of thinly sliced ham. Cut the ham slices in half and wrap them around the curd. The ham is sticky enough to stick to the cheese without a toothpick. Continue with the recipe as described above.

Nutritional information (per serving)

calories 317

fats 27.5 g 78%

proteins 10.9 g 13%

carbohydrates 7.6 g 9%

fibers 0,6 g

Cheese nachos

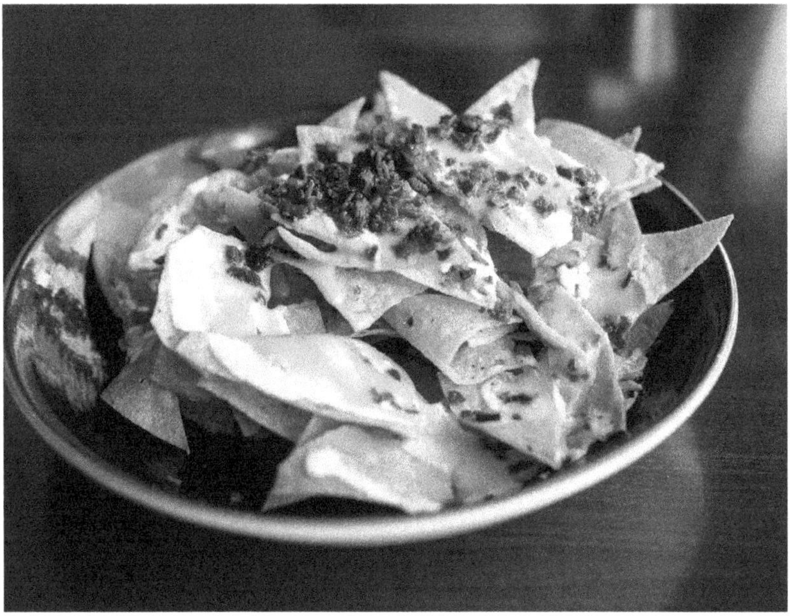

KETO - WITHOUT NUTS

Preparation time: 10 minutes

Cooking time: 30 minutes

Yield: 6 servings

½ cup grated extra-sharp cheddar cheese (about 60 grams), frozen

3 large egg whites

⅛ teaspoon of cream tartare

2 teaspoons of taco seasoning

NECESSARY MATERIAL

KITCHEN ROBOT

1. Preheat the oven to 150 ° C. Line a baking sheet with parchment paper.

2. Place the frozen grated cheese in a food processor and cut into small pieces.

3. In a bowl, beat the egg whites with the cream of tartar until very stiff peaks form. Sprinkle the chopped frozen cheese over the whites. Then, with a rubber spatula, very carefully fold the cheese into the egg whites, making sure not to disturb the fluffy whites while still spreading the cheese completely.

4. Carefully place the mixture in a large sealable plastic bag, then cut a 1cm hole in the corner of the bag. Gently squeeze the mixture onto the prepared pan into strips about 6cm long and 1cm wide. Lightly sprinkle the top of each pastry with the taco dressing.

5. Cook for 20-30 minutes. The longer you can cook them, the crisper they will be, but don't let them get too brown. For even more crunchy puffs, turn off the oven and leave them in the oven for at least another 30 minutes.

6. Store in an airtight airtight container for up to 7 days. It is eaten fresh.

Nutritional information (per serving)

calories 57

fat 3,5 g 55%

protein 4,6 g 32%

carbohydrates 1,8 g 13%

fibers 0.7 g

Condiments

Slow cooker bone broth

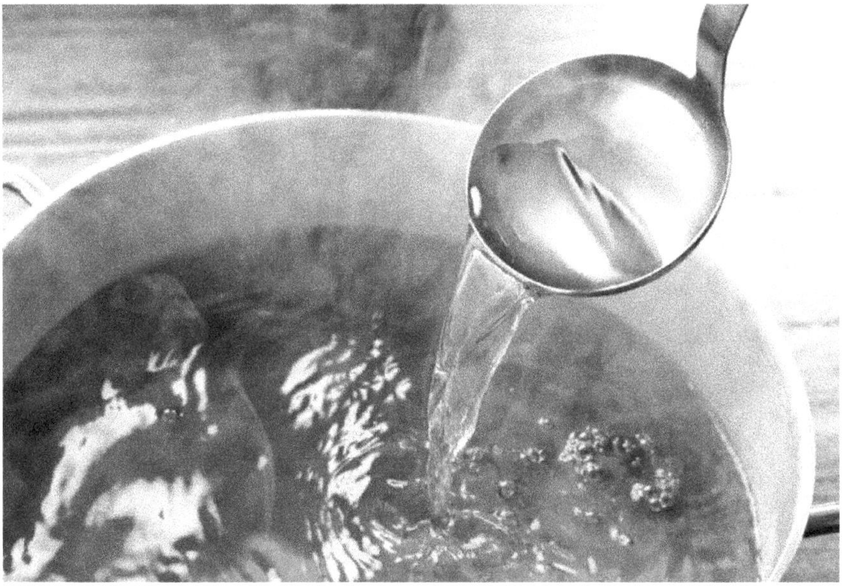

KETO - WITHOUT NUTS - WITHOUT LACTOSE

Preparation time: 12 minutes

Cooking time: 1 to 2 days

Yield: 4 quarts (1 cup per serving)

When making bone broth, using an acid such as organic vinegar helps extract more minerals from the bones. The extracted minerals, in turn, neutralize the acidity of the vinegar, so it does not affect the overall flavor of the broth. I use coconut vinegar, which surpasses all other vinegars in amino acid, vitamin and mineral content. It is also a prebiotic that promotes digestive health. Don't worry, it doesn't taste like coconut!

1 ½ kg of beef, chicken, ham or fish bones

2 celery sticks, chopped

1 medium yellow onion, chopped

7 cloves of garlic, crushed with the side of a knife

2 bay leaves

2 teaspoons of fine sea salt

¼ cup of coconut vinegar

Cold filtered water

¼ cup fresh herbs or 1 teaspoon dried herbs of your choice (optional)

Necessary material

STOVE on SLOW heat - COLINO

Variation

Vegetable broth. For a vegetarian broth, simply omit the bones. You can also add more vegetables, such as carrots and leeks.

Tip for busy families

Prepare a huge batch and store the portions in glass jars in the freezer for easy use in recipes.

1. Place the bones, vegetables, garlic, bay leaves, salt and coconut vinegar in a 6-quart slow cooker and add enough cold filtered water to cover everything.

2. Add your favorite herbs, if you use them.

3. Set the slow cooker to high heat and cook for about 30 minutes, then reduce the heat to low. Remove any foam or scum that appears on the surface.

4. Cook over low heat for 1 to 2 days. The long cooking time allows you to extract more gelatin and minerals from the bones. When the broth is ready, pour it into a colander and remove the solids.

5. The broth will keep in the fridge for about 5 days or in the freezer for several months. When needed for recipes or a cup of healing broth, pour the meaty substance into a cup and heat it to make it a nice thick liquid again.

Nutritional information (per serving)

calories 13

fat 0 g 0%

protein 1,5 g 46%

carbohydrates 1.7 g 52%

fibers 0 g

Tips for making the best bone broth

1. Roast beef, lamb, pork and chicken bones in advance. Why? It adds color and flavor. Roast the large bones at 190 ° C for 50-60 minutes, the smaller bones for 30-40 minutes.

2. Start by covering the roasted bones with cold filtered water. Why? Some proteins, especially albumin, will only dissolve in cold water. Albumin helps clarify the broth, so if you start with cold water, you'll end up with a nice clear broth. And since a substantial part of broth preparation comes down to getting rid of impurities, it makes sense to start with the purest water you can use.

3. Don't skip the vinegar. Why? It extracts minerals from the bones.

4. Use crow's feet to make chicken bone broth. Why? They add more collagen and create a denser broth.

5. Add your favorite herbs. Not only do they add flavor, but they also add nutrition. Rosemary, in particular, helps to extract extra calcium from the bones.

6. Save the remaining bones. Whenever you make beef, chicken, or fish dishes, store the remaining bones in the freezer until you have enough bones and time to make broth.

Why bone broth?

From a culinary point of view, bone broth is superior to store-bought chicken or beef broth. It has the best flavor and the collagen leaking out of the bones makes it a natural thickener, ideal for creating pleasant and thick sauces. If you substitute a store-bought broth in these recipes, you probably won't get a thick consistency.

From a health perspective, bone broth is beyond compare. It's incredibly nutritious and so good for you that if it could be sold in pill form, the drug companies would go broke. Its medicinal benefits are attributed to the exceptionally high levels of minerals and amino acids it gets from the bones. In fact, bone broth can be considered a high quality mineral and protein supplement. Here are some of the most notable benefits of bone broth.

1. Attracts digestive juices: The gelatin in bone broth is a hydrophilic colloid, which is an elegant way of saying it attracts liquids. This is important because it means it attracts digestive juices for quick and effective digestion.

2. Heals the gut: The gelatin in the broth works surprisingly well as a treatment for intestinal ailments, including hyperacidity, colitis and Crohn's disease because it helps heal the intestinal wall and its many nutrients are easily absorbed, which can be a problem with these ailments. It also helps many people digest dairy products more easily, and strengthening the intestinal wall also supports the immune system. Bone broth should be the first therapeutic food for those suffering from digestive disorders affecting the intestine.

3. Helps cure other diseases: Jelly in bone broth is also useful for treating anemia, diabetes, muscular dystrophy and even cancer.

4. Increases Protein Absorption: Although gelatin is not a complete protein (it only contains the amino acids arginine and glycine in large quantities), it allows the body to make full use of the complete proteins that are consumed. If you can't afford large amounts of meat in your diet, gelatin-rich broths are a great way to boost protein absorption.

5. Contains Many Minerals: Healthy bone tissue is naturally rich in calcium, magnesium, phosphorus and potassium, which are necessary for a healthy bone structure, nervous system and hormonal balance. Fish bone broths also contain iodine, which is essential for a healthy thyroid.

6. Improves Joint Health: Because gelatin is derived from cartilage, bone broth is an excellent source of glucosamine and chondroitin, essential nutrients for joint health.

"Buttery" compound

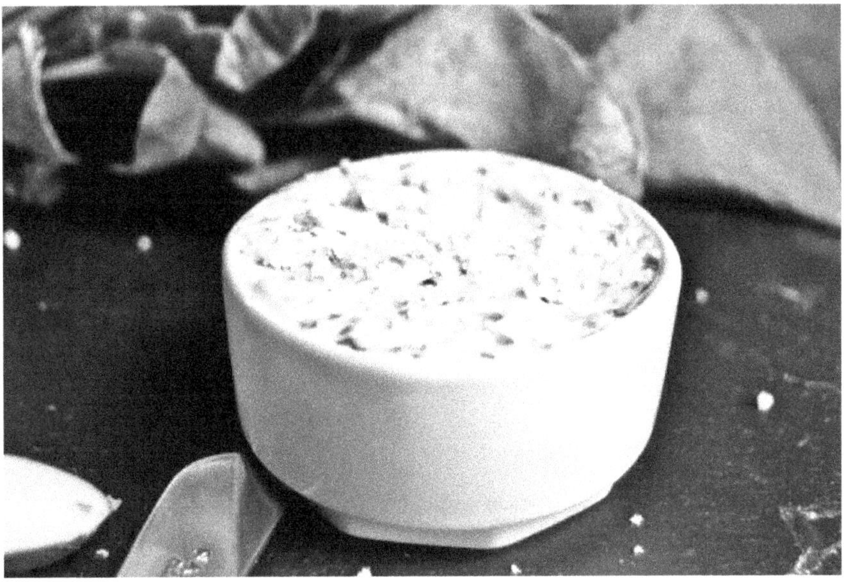

KETO - WITHOUT NUTS - WITHOUT LACTOSE

Preparation time: 8 minutes, plus 3 hours to chill

Yield: 1 cup (1 tablespoon per serving)

Many times when I ask customers to cut out their dairy, they can't imagine a life without butter. Using healthy natural animal fats, like beef tallow and duck fat, is a great way to add flavor and satisfy cravings for that creamy and buttery texture. This "buttery" compound tastes great on grilled vegetables and meats. I also like to give it away!

You are invited to mix the flavors of "butter" using your favorite flavor profiles.

½ cup of beef tallow or leaf lard, softened

½ cup of duck fat, softened

1 head of roasted garlic

1 tablespoon of finely chopped fresh rosemary

1 tablespoon finely chopped fresh oregano

1 tablespoon finely chopped fresh chives

Fine sea salt and freshly ground black pepper to taste

1. In a medium-sized bowl, mix all the ingredients. Place the mixture on a sheet of parchment paper. Roll into a log shape and twist the ends of the paper to seal.

2. Refrigerate the "butter" until it hardens, about 3 hours. Cut into coins to serve.

Note

Mix beef tallow (or leaf lard) and duck fat because at room temperature, beef tallow and leaf lard are very solid while duck fat is almost liquid. Together they give an amazing flavor and buttery texture. If you're not sensitive to dairy, you can use 1 cup unsalted butter at room temperature instead of beef tallow and duck fat.

Variations

Although the recipe above is my favorite flavor of "butter", I have tried many combinations over the years, all of which are delicious. If you are looking for new flavor combinations, try the following:

• 1 tablespoon of finely chopped fresh rosemary, finely chopped fresh mint and grated lemon zest

• 1 tablespoon each of finely chopped fresh coriander, grated lime zest and ground cumin

• 1 tablespoon each of finely chopped fresh thyme, finely chopped fresh rosemary and finely chopped fresh sage

• 1 tablespoon each of finely chopped fresh lemongrass and turmeric powder

• 1 tablespoon of finely chopped fresh lemongrass, finely chopped fresh tarragon and Dijon mustard

Nutritional information (per serving)

calories 123

fat 13 g 95%

protein 0.2 g 1%

carbohydrates 1,4 g 4%

fibers 0 g

Roasted garlic

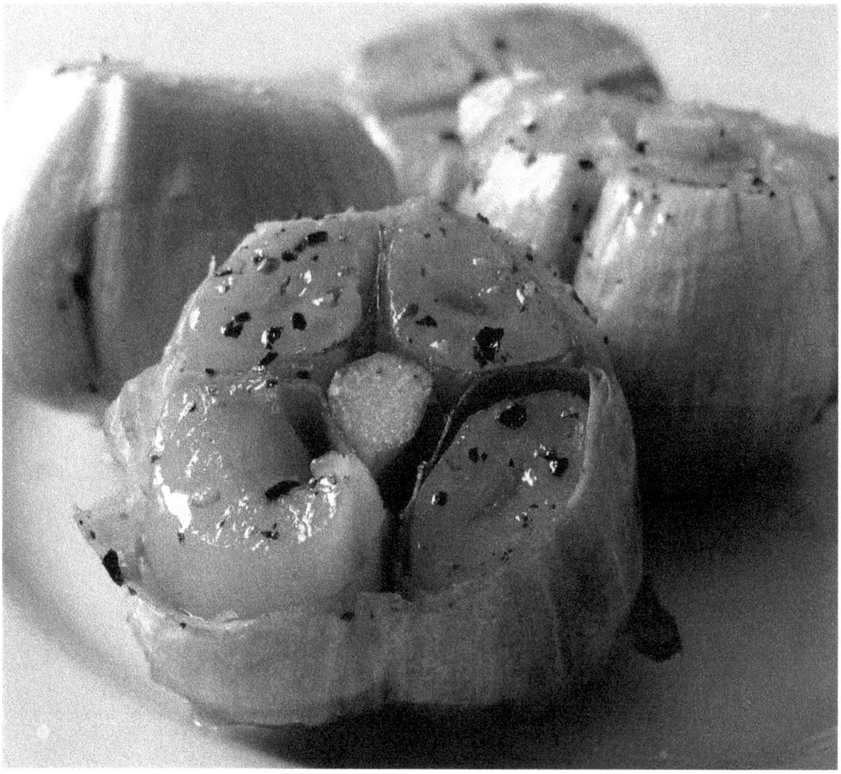

KETO - WITHOUT NUTS - WITHOUT LACTOSE

Preparation time: 5 minutes

Cooking time: 40 minutes

Yield: 12 people

12 heads of garlic

¼ cup of MCT oil

½ teaspoon of fine sea salt

Tip for busy families

Always keep roasted garlic in the freezer for easy use in recipes.

1. Preheat the oven to 180 degrees.

2. Cut some of the top of the garlic to expose the cloves and place the garlic in a pan. Pour the MCT oil over the tops of the garlic heads, letting the oil soak into the cloves and sprinkle the tops with salt. Cover the pan with aluminum foil and place in the oven to cook.

3. The garlic is ready when a central clove is completely soft when pierced with a kitchen knife. Even after it's soft, you can continue toasting until deep brown for a more caramelized flavor - check the garlic every 10 minutes. The exact roasting time will depend on the size of your garlic head, the variety and its age.

4. Allow to cool and squeeze the garlic cloves from the skins as needed. Store unused roasted garlic in the skin in the freezer for up to 3 months.

Nutritional information (per person)

calories 97

fats 4. 8 g 45%

protein 2.3 g 9%

carbohydrates 11.5 g 47%

fibers 0. 8 g

Dutch - dairy free

KETO - WITHOUT NUTS - WITHOUT LACTOSE

Preparation time: 5 minutes

Cooking time: 5 minutes

Yield: 2 cups (about 2 and a half tablespoons per serving)

6 large egg yolks

¼ cup of lemon juice

2 tablespoons of mustard

1 1/2 cups bacon fat, lard or duck fat, melted (but not too hot)

½ teaspoon of cayenne pepper

½ teaspoon of fine sea salt

⅛ teaspoon of freshly ground black pepper

1. At the bottom of a double boiler or in a medium-sized saucepan, bring one inch of water to a boil over high heat, then adjust the heat to keep it boiling. Place the egg yolks, lemon juice, and mustard in the top of the double boiler or in a heat resistant bowl that fits into the saucepan with the boiling water.

2. Beat the yolk mixture to combine, then, stirring constantly, add the melted fat in a slow, steady stream (this should take about 90 seconds). Cook the sauce, beating, until it reaches 60 ° C.

3. Add the cayenne pepper, salt and pepper and continue whisking until thick, about 3 minutes, adjusting the heat to

maintain a temperature of 60 ° C (remove from the boiling water if necessary). Adjust the toppings to taste.

Variation: Traditional Dutch

If you're not sensitive to dairy, use unsalted melted butter as fat (in place of bacon fat, lard, or duck fat) to create a traditional hollandaise sauce.

Nutritional information (per serving)

calories 241

fat 26 g 97%

proteins 1,4 g 2%

carbohydrates 0,6 g 1%

fibers 0 g

Homemade mustard

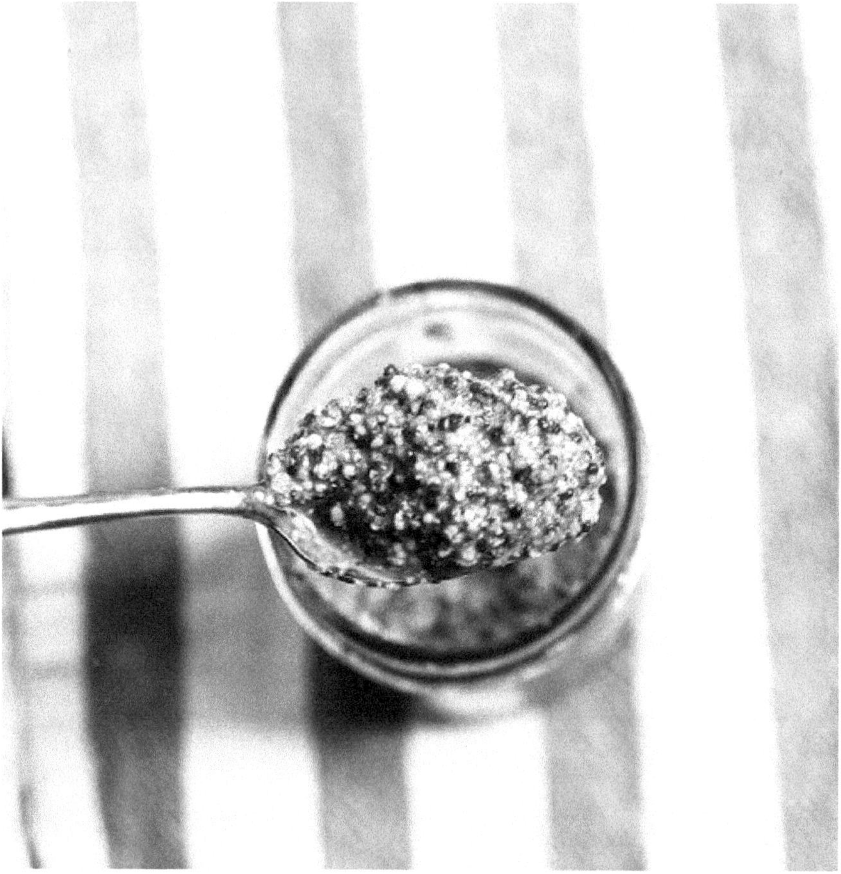

KETO - WITHOUT NUTS - WITHOUT LACTOSE

Preparation time: 5 minutes, plus 8 hours to chill

Yield: 1 cup (about 1 tablespoon per serving)

Mustard seeds or mustard powder? It's a bit like asking, "Do you like crunchy or creamy peanut butter?"

I suggest using seeds when you want a crunchy texture. Keep in mind that darker seeds have a much stronger flavor.

There are three types of seeds:

• Yellow, also known as white, which has the mildest flavor. They are mainly used in American mustard and for pickling.
• Brown, which is a little spicier than yellow and is used in European-style mustards (such as Dijon) and for pickling when a deeper flavor is desired. They are also used in Indian cooking.

• Black, which tastes similar to brown seeds and is also used in Indian cooking.

If you decide to make mustard from seeds, you need to soften them in a liquid for 1 or 2 days in advance.

I suggest using mustard powder if you want a silky smooth mustard. Mustard powder is made from finely ground white and brown mustard seeds. If you use the powder, all you need to do is mix it with a liquid (like water or bone broth ... not beer!) And let it sit overnight to fully hydrate and develop flavor. Don't let it sit any longer, though, or it will taste tart.

⅓ cup of coconut vinegar or apple cider vinegar

⅓ cup of white wine vinegar

⅓ cup of powdered erythritol

3 tablespoons of yellow mustard seeds

2 ½ tablespoons of brown mustard seeds

2 tablespoons of chopped shallots

¾ teaspoon of fine sea salt

¼ teaspoon of ground white pepper

1/4 teaspoon fish sauce (optional; for umami)

A pinch of ground allspice

Necessary material

MIXER

Tip: To make the mustard more keto, I like to add a few tablespoons of brown butter

Sweet and spicy mustard

1. In a medium-sized glass or non-reactive metal bowl, combine all ingredients, cover and refrigerate overnight.

2. Transfer the mixture to a blender and blend until the mustard has the desired consistency and thickness. I prefer to keep it chunky, but you can make it smooth if you prefer.

3. Store in the refrigerator in an airtight glass container for up to 2 weeks.

Nutritional information (per serving)

calories 21

fats 1.1 g 47%

protein 1 g 19%

carbohydrates 1.7 g 32%

fibers 0,6 g

Dijon mustard

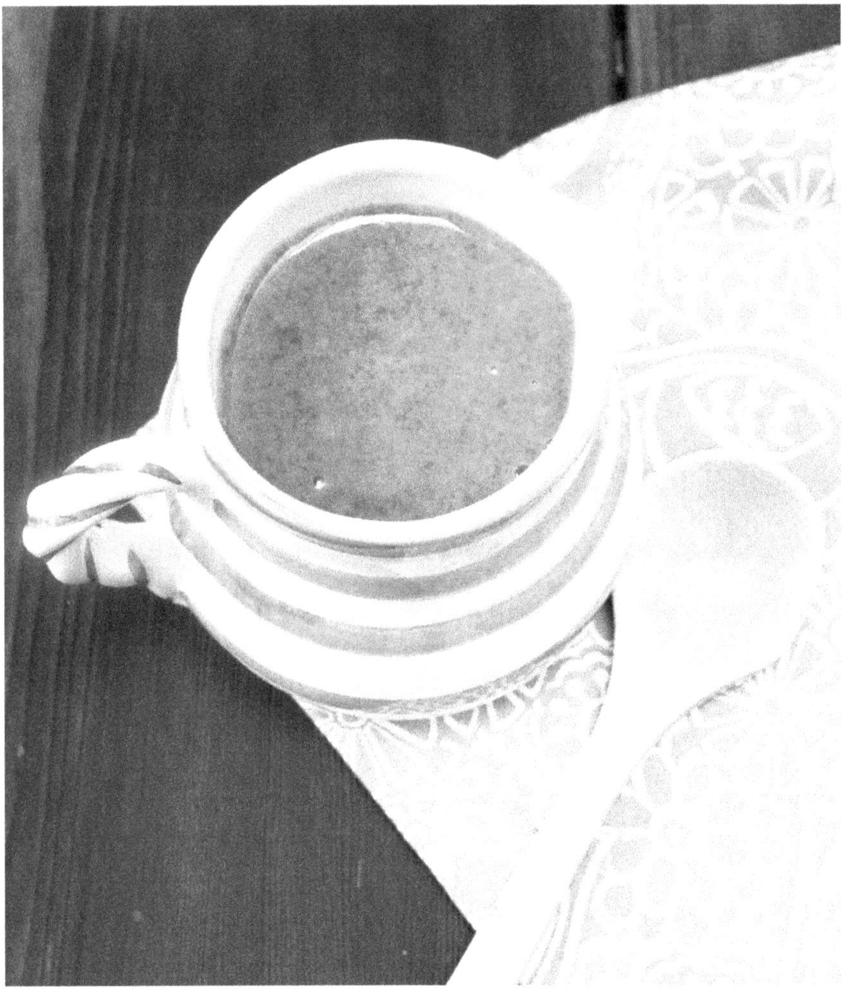

KETO - WITHOUT NUTS - WITHOUT LACTOSE

Preparation time: 5 minutes, plus 2 days to cool

Yield: 1 cup (about 1 tablespoon per serving)

⅓ cup of brown mustard seeds

⅓ cup of white wine vinegar

⅓ cup of beef bone broth, plus more if needed

1 tablespoon of powdered erythritol

1 tsp ground turmeric

½ teaspoon of fine sea salt

⅛ teaspoon of cayenne pepper

⅛ teaspoon of stevia glycerite

1 or 2 teaspoons of prepared horseradish (optional)

1. In a medium-sized glass or non-reactive metal bowl, combine all ingredients except the horseradish. Cover and refrigerate for 2 days.

2. Transfer the mixture to a blender and blend until the mustard is as smooth as desired. Add 2-4 tablespoons of beef broth if the mustard is too thick.

3. If you prefer a spicy mustard, add the horseradish.

4. Store in the refrigerator for up to 1 month.

Necessary material

MIXER

Nutritional information (per serving)

calories 18

fat 1 g 50%

protein 0.9 g 20%

carbohydrates 1,4 g 31%

fibers 0.5 g

Thyme mustard with rosemary

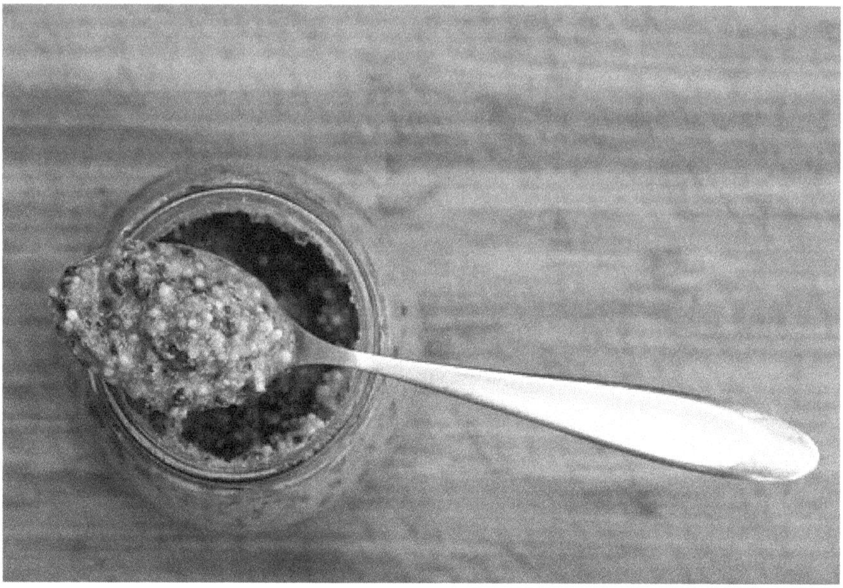

KETO - WITHOUT NUTS - WITHOUT LACTOSE

Preparation time: 5 minutes, plus 2 days to cool

Yield: 1 cup (about 1 tablespoon per serving)

⅓ cup of water or beef bone broth

⅓ cup of coconut vinegar or apple cider vinegar

3 tablespoons of yellow mustard seeds

1 tablespoon of brown mustard seeds

1 tablespoon of powdered erythritol or ⅛ teaspoon of stevia glycerite

2 teaspoons of chopped fresh thyme

2 teaspoons of chopped fresh rosemary

¾ teaspoon of fine sea salt

1/4 teaspoon fish sauce (optional; for umami)

1. In a medium-sized glass or non-reactive metal bowl, combine all the ingredients. Cover and refrigerate for 2 days.

2. Put the mixture in a blender and whisk until the mustard is thick but still coarse.

3. Store in the refrigerator for up to 1 month.

Necessary material

MIXER

Nutritional information (per serving)

calories 15

fat 0,8 g 48%

protein 0.7 g 19%

carbohydrates 1.2 g 32%

fibers 0.5 g

BBQ mustard

Preparation time: 5 minutes, plus 8 hours to chill

Cooking time: 40 minutes

Yield: 2 cups (about 1 tablespoon per serving)

1 cup sweet and spicy mustard or other prepared yellow mustard¼ cup of powdered erythritol or ¼ teaspoon of stevia glycerite

¾ cup of coconut vinegar or apple cider vinegar

1 tablespoon of chili powder

1 teaspoon of freshly ground black pepper

1 teaspoon of ground white pepper

¼ teaspoon of cayenne pepper

½ teaspoon of tamari or coconut without grain aminos

2 tablespoons unsalted butter or coconut oil

1 teaspoon of liquid smoke

1. In a saucepan over medium heat, mix the mustard, erythritol, vinegar, chili powder, black pepper, white pepper, and cayenne pepper. Boil for 30 minutes.

2. Incorporate the tamari, butter and liquid smoke and simmer for another 10 minutes. Let it cool completely and transfer to a glass jar. Refrigerate overnight to blend the flavors before use.

3. Store in the refrigerator for up to 4 weeks.

Nutritional information (per serving)

calories 19.5

fat 1,4 g 62%

proteins 0,6 g 12%

carbohydrates 1.2 g 24%

fibers 0.3 g

Tartar sauce

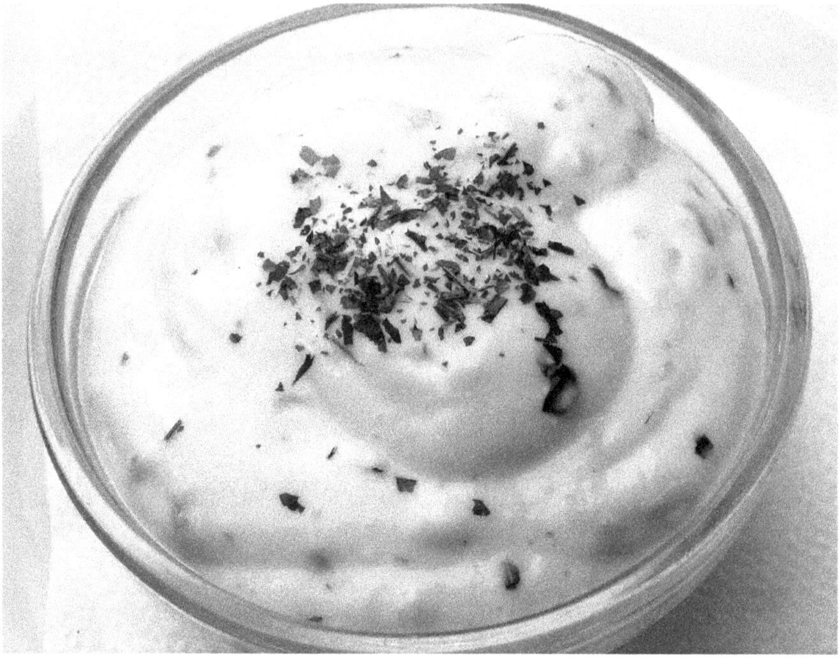

KETO - WITHOUT NUTS - WITHOUT LACTOSE

Preparation time: 5 minutes

Yield: ¾ cup (2 tablespoons per serving)

Put all the ingredients in a food processor and blend until well combined but not yet blended. Store in an airtight container in the refrigerator for up to 2 weeks.

½ cup of mayonnaise

2 tablespoons finely diced dill pickles

1 tablespoon of coconut vinegar or white wine vinegar

¼ teaspoon of fine sea salt

⅛ teaspoon of freshly ground black pepper

Necessary material

KITCHEN ROBOT

Nutritional information (per serving)

calories 121

fats 13.3 g 99%

protein 0 g 0%

carbohydrates 0.5 g 2%

fibers 0 g

"Honey" dressing

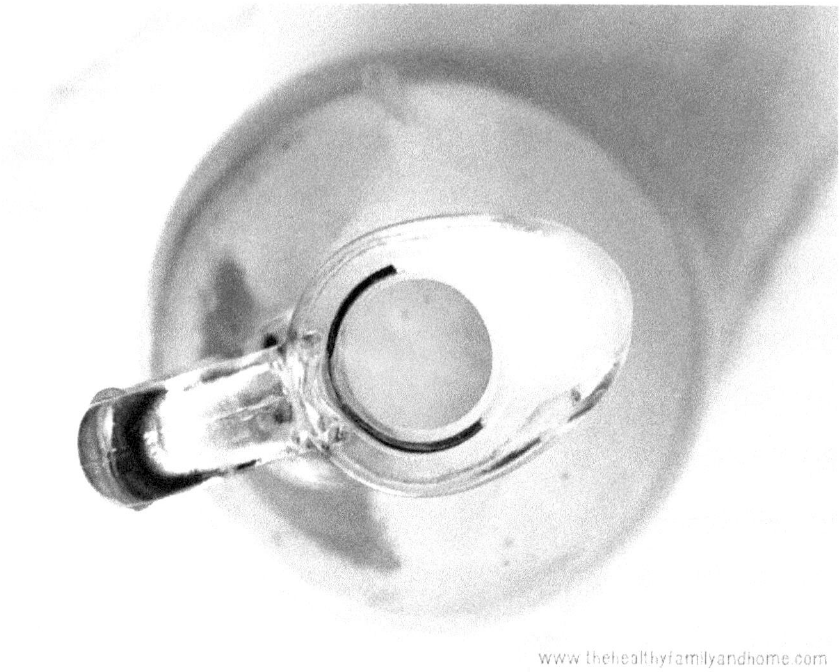

KETO

Preparation time: 2 minutes

Cooking time: 15 minutes

Yield: 1 1/2 cups (2 tablespoons per serving)

Before you start, make sure you have everything ready. You have to work fast or the sweetener will burn.

½ cup (1 stick) of unsalted butter

30 grams of cream cheese (about 2 tablespoons)

¼ cup of powdered erythritol

½ cup of unsweetened almond milk

1. In a heavy-bottomed 2- or 3-quart saucepan, heat the butter over high heat. As soon as it comes to a boil, watch over the brown specks (this is brown butter, so good with vegetables!). Immediately add the cream cheese and blend until smooth and without cream cheese pieces.

2. Add erythritol and almond milk and whisk until smooth. Let it cool in the pan for a couple of minutes, then pour it into a glass jar and let it cool to room temperature.

3. Store in the refrigerator for up to 2 weeks. To reheat, place in a small saucepan and heat over low heat for a minute, until liquefied.

Nutritional information (per serving)

calories 78

fat 8,5 g 98%

protein 0.3 g 2%

carbohydrates 0.1 g 1%

fibers 0 g

Lactose-free avocado dressing

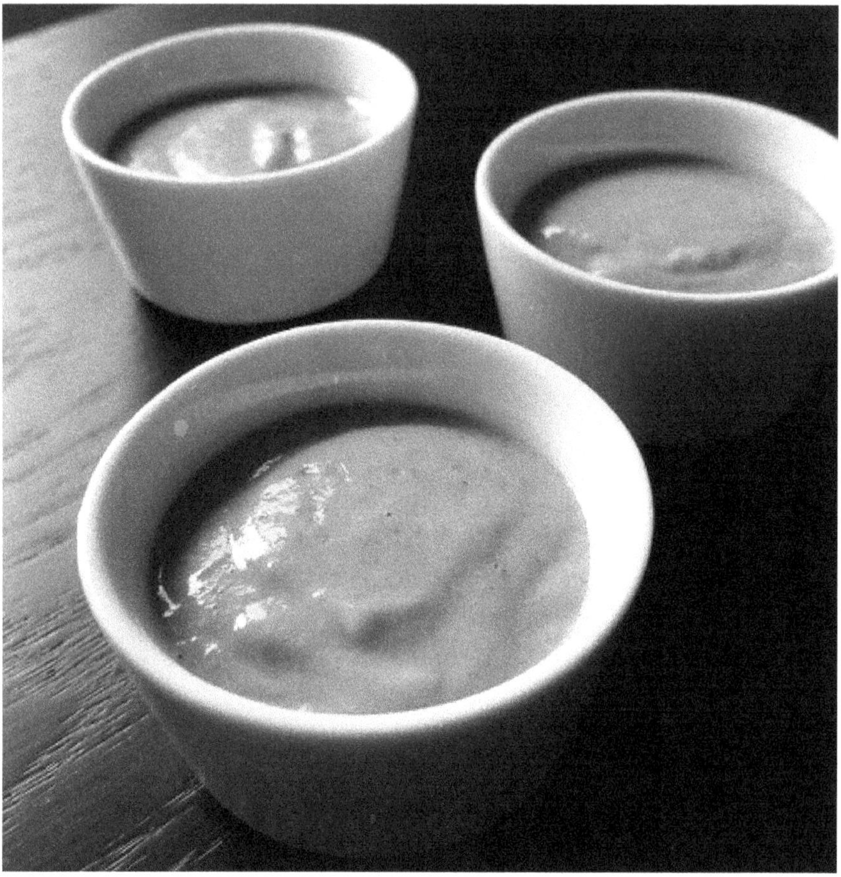

KETO - WITHOUT NUTS - WITHOUT LACTOSE

Preparation time: 5 minutes

Yield: 2 cups (2 tablespoons per serving)

Put all the ingredients in a blender or food processor and blend until smooth. Add more broth to dilute the dressing if desired. Place in a glass jar, cover and refrigerate for up to 2 weeks.

1 avocado, cut in half and pitted

1 head of roasted garlic

½ cup of chicken or beef bone broth

½ cup of or mayonnaise

2 tablespoons chopped fresh flat-leaf parsley

2 tablespoons of chopped fresh dill

½ teaspoon of coconut vinegar

½ teaspoon of smoked paprika

¼ teaspoon of onion powder

¼ teaspoon of fine sea salt

¼ teaspoon of freshly ground black pepper

½ tsp fish sauce (optional; for umami)

Necessary material

BLENDER or KITCHEN ROBOT

Nutritional information (per serving)

calories 86

fat 8 g

proteins 1.8 g 82%

carbohydrates 2.6 g 8%

fiber 1.1 g 11%

Ranch dressing

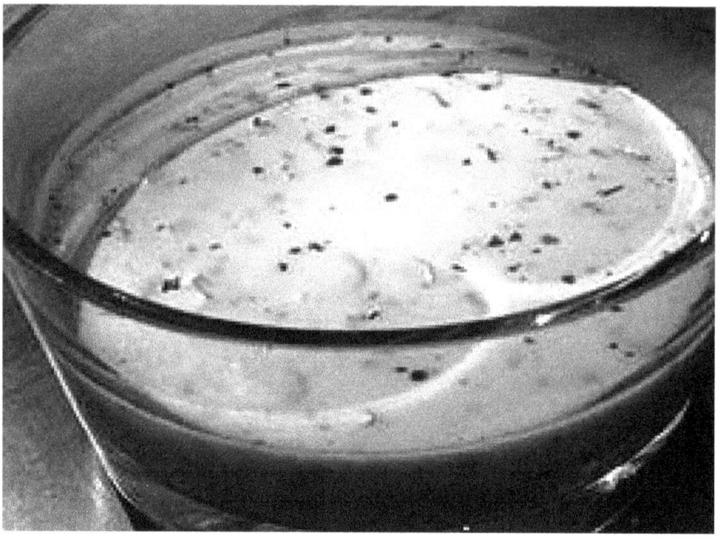

KETO - WITHOUT NUTS

Preparation time: 5 minutes, plus 2 hours to chill

Yield: 1 1/2 cups (2 tablespoons per serving)

In a blender or large bowl, mix all the ingredients. Transfer to a glass jar, cover and refrigerate for 2 hours before serving (it will thicken as it rests). Store in the refrigerator for up to 2 weeks.

220 grams of cream cheese (about 1 cup), softened

½ cup of chicken or beef bone broth

½ teaspoon of dried chives

½ teaspoon of dried parsley

½ teaspoon of dried dill herb

¼ teaspoon of garlic powder

¼ teaspoon of onion powder

⅛ teaspoon of fine sea salt

⅛ teaspoon of freshly ground black pepper

Necessary material

MIXER

Nutritional information (per serving)

calories 69

fats 6.6 g 86%

proteins 1.7 g 10%

carbohydrates 0.7 g 4%

fibers 0 g

Thousand island sauce - lactose free

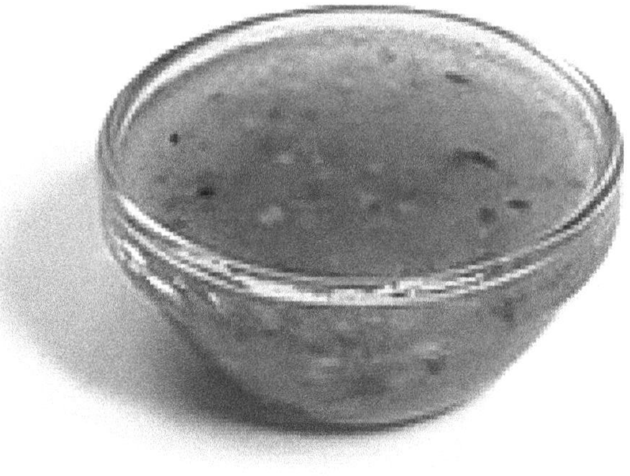

KETO - WITHOUT NUTS - WITHOUT LACTOSE

Preparation time: 2 minutes

Yield: 1 ¼ cups (2 tablespoons per serving)

Put all the ingredients in a jar and shake well. Store in the refrigerator for up to 2 weeks.

¾ cup of mayonnaise

1/4 cup chopped dill pickles

¼ cup of tomato sauce, homemade or store-bought

2 tablespoons of powdered erythritol or a drop of stevia glycerite

⅛ teaspoon of fine sea salt

⅛ teaspoon of fish sauce

Nutritional information (per serving)

calories 59

fat 4,9 g 75%

protein 0.2 g 1%

carbohydrates 3.8 g 24%

fibers 1.2 g

Fat-burning salad dressing

KETO - WITHOUT NUTS - WITHOUT LACTOSE

Preparation time: 2 minutes

Yield: ¾ cup (2 tablespoons per serving)

This is a great way to add fat to a meal - just sprinkle.

Put all the ingredients in a jar and shake well. Store in the refrigerator for up to 6 weeks.

½ cup of MCT oil

¼ cup of coconut vinegar or apple cider vinegar

1 teaspoon of fine sea salt

½ teaspoon of freshly ground black pepper

½ teaspoon of stevia glycerite

½ teaspoon of fish sauce

Nutritional information (per serving)

174 calories

fats 18.7 g 98%

proteins 0.1 g 1%

carbohydrates 0.1 g 1%

fibers 0 g

Greek salad dressing

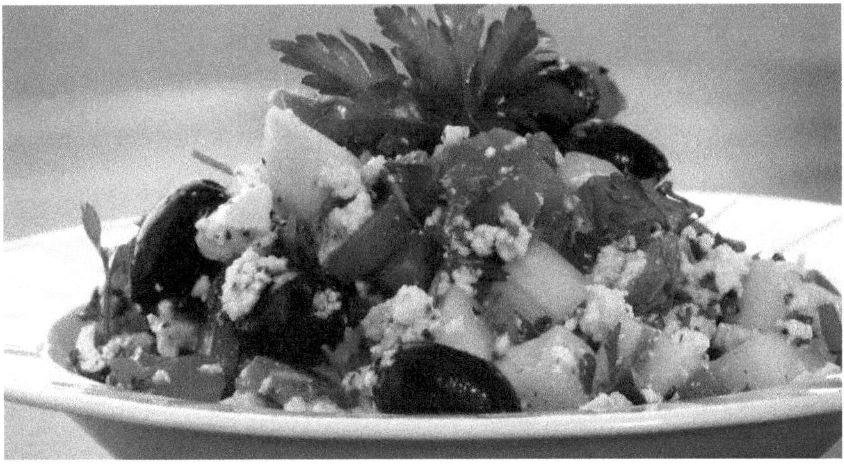

KETO - WITHOUT NUTS - WITHOUT LACTOSE

Preparation time: 8 minutes

Yield: ½ cup (2 tablespoons per serving)

Juice of 1 lemon or lime

¼ cup of MCT oil

1 clove of garlic, minced

2 tablespoons of finely chopped fresh oregano

1 tablespoon of finely chopped fresh basil

½ teaspoon of fine sea salt

½ teaspoon of freshly ground black pepper

⅛ teaspoon of fish sauce (optional; for umami)

1. Put the lemon juice, MCT oil, garlic, oregano and basil in a blender or food processor. Stir to mix well. Add salt, pepper and fish sauce, if used, and whisk to combine.

2. Store in a glass jar in the refrigerator for up to 2 weeks.

Necessary material

BLENDER or KITCHEN ROBOT

Nutritional information (per serving)

calories 139

fat 14.3 g 93%

proteins 0.5 g 1%

carbohydrates 2.1 g 6%

fibers 1.1 g

Tomato sauce

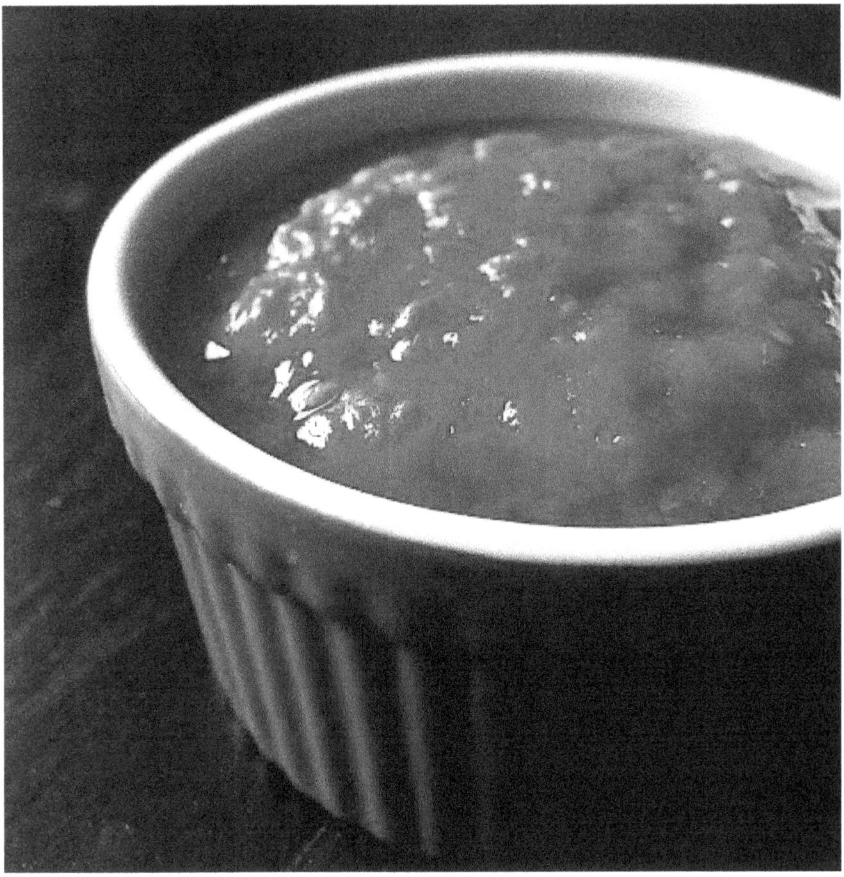

KETO - WITHOUT NUTS - WITHOUT LACTOSE

Preparation time: 10 minutes

Cooking time: 25 minutes

Yield: About 2 cups (1/4 cup per serving)

2 tablespoons of MCT oil

1/2 cup diced yellow onion

1 roasted head of garlic or 3 cloves of raw garlic, minced

2 large tomatoes, pureed (about 2 cups)

¼ cup of chopped fresh basil

1/4 teaspoon stevia glycerite (optional)

½ teaspoon of fine sea salt

⅛ teaspoon of freshly ground black pepper

1. Heat the MCT oil in a large saucepan over medium-high heat. Add the onion and garlic and cook until the onion turns translucent and begins to brown, stirring often.

2. Add the rest of the ingredients and simmer until the sauce thickens and covers a tablespoon, about 20 minutes.

Variation: pizza sauce

To turn it into pizza sauce, simmer for another 30 minutes to thicken it further and then whisk it in a blender until smooth.

Nutritional information (per serving)

calories 46

fats 3.6 g 70%

proteins 0,6 g 5%

carbohydrates 2.9 g 25%

fibers 0.7 g

Yellow marinara sauce

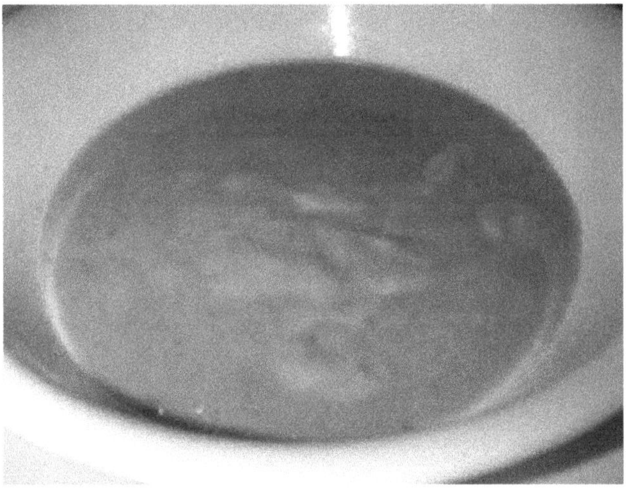

KETO - WITHOUT NUTS - WITHOUT LACTOSE

Preparation time: 5 minutes

Cooking time: 3 and a half hours

Yield: 2 quarts (about ⅓ cup per serving)

A great tomato sauce has a balance of sweetness and acidity, but making the perfect sauce can be difficult. This recipe uses a couple of tricks to counteract the natural acidity of tomatoes, starting with the choice of tomatoes: yellow tomatoes are less acidic than red tomatoes. Plus, taking the time to caramelize the onions creates a natural sweetness that helps balance the sour taste.

2.2 kg of yellow tomatoes

1/4 cup beef tallow or coconut oil (or unsalted butter if not sensitive to dairy)

1 cup diced yellow onion

1 teaspoon plus 1 pinch of fine sea salt

1 cup of sliced champignon mushrooms (see note)

2 heads of roasted garlic or 8 cloves of raw garlic, minced

⅓ cup of finely chopped fresh basil

2 sprigs of fresh flat-leaf parsley or 1 tsp dried

1 sprig of fresh oregano or 1 tsp dried

1 sprig of fresh thyme or ½ tsp dried

2 bay leaves

2 teaspoons of red pepper flakes (optional)

½ teaspoon of stevia glycerite (optional)

NOTE: Butter cuts the sour taste of tomatoes, as well as mushrooms.

1. Bring a large pot of water to a boil. Prepare an ice bath in a large bowl.

2. Cut a small "X" on top of each tomato and drop them into the boiling water, a few at a time, for 10 seconds. Remove with a slotted spoon and drop into the ice bath. Peel the tomatoes (the skin will peel off easily) and cut them into quarters. Remove the seeds with a teaspoon and coarsely chop the tomato quarters.

3. Place the beef tallow in a large pot over medium heat. Add the onion and sauté for 15-20 minutes, until the onion turns dark brown, stirring often to prevent burning. Add a pinch of salt to the onion as it cooks. (This speeds up the caramelizing process; the salt sucks the moisture from the onion.) Keep stirring and watch as the onion gets darker and darker. If you feel the onions sticking too much to the bottom of the pan,

add a very small amount of water or broth and stir vigorously to deglaze the pan.

4. Add the mushrooms and garlic to the caramelized onions and saute for 8 minutes or until the mushrooms are tender. Add the tomatoes, the aromatic herbs (leave the fresh twigs whole), the red pepper flakes, if used, and 1 teaspoon of salt. Simmer over low heat for 2 to 3 hours, or until cooked through and starting to darken. Remove the sprigs of aromatic herbs and bay leaves. If you wish, add stevia.

5. Optional: Use a hand blender to blend the sauce until smooth. For a thicker sauce, skip this step.

6. Store in the refrigerator for up to 7 days, or can according to the conservator's instructions for tomato-based products. Just before serving, add some flavor enhancers if desired.

Optional flavor enhancers and acid neutralizers

Whipped cream: add a splash and let the sauce cook for a few minutes to thicken.

Hard Cheeses: Add ½ cup of grated Parmesan, pecorino or other hard cheese to give the sauce a deep savory note.

Fresh cheeses and other fermented dairy products: Add a dollop of mascarpone, cream cheese, or crème fraîche.

Nutritional information (per serving)

calories 48

fats 2,5 g 47%

protein 0.9 g 8%

carbohydrates 5.5 g 46%

fibers 0.9 g

Keto ketchup

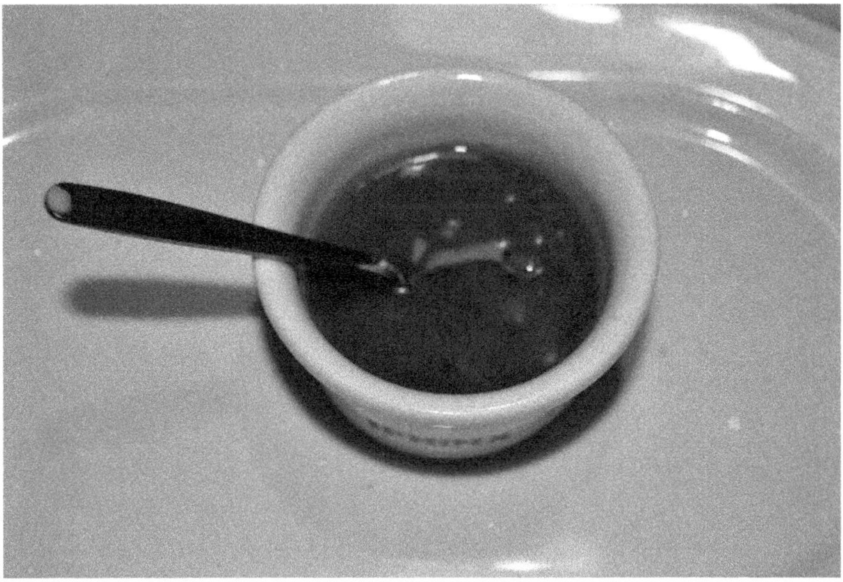

KETO - WITHOUT NUTS - WITHOUT LACTOSE

Preparation time: 2 minutes

Cooking time: 45 minutes

Yield: 2 cups (2 tablespoons per serving)

1 ½ cup of beef or chicken broth or water

1 jar of tomato paste

2 tablespoons of apple cider vinegar or coconut vinegar

1 tablespoon of powdered erythritol or 1 drop of stevia glycerite

1 teaspoon of garlic powder

1 teaspoon of onion powder

1 teaspoon of fine sea salt

1. Combine all ingredients in a medium sized saucepan. Bring to a boil, then reduce the heat and simmer for 45 minutes.

2. Store in an airtight container in the refrigerator for up to 2 weeks.

Nutritional information (per serving)

calories 17

fats 0.2 g 11%

protein 1 g 24%

carbohydrates 2.7 g 64%

fibers 0.5 g

Keto barbecue sauce

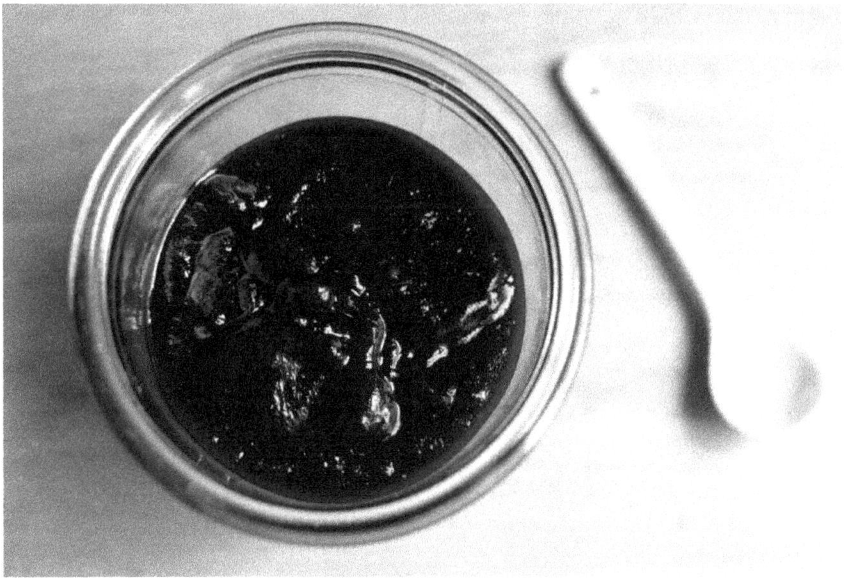

KETO - WITHOUT NUTS - WITHOUT LACTOSE

Preparation time: 3 minutes

Yield: 2 ½ cups (about 1 ½ tablespoons per serving)

Put all the ingredients in a large bowl and mix well. Store in an airtight container in the refrigerator for up to 2 weeks.

2 cups of Chetto Ketchup

¼ cup of powdered erythritol or 1 teaspoon of stevia glycerite

2 tablespoons of coconut vinegar or apple cider vinegar

1 and a half teaspoons of liquid smoke

½ teaspoon of onion powder

½ teaspoon of garlic powder

½ teaspoon of freshly ground black pepper

⅛ teaspoon of fine sea salt

Nutritional information (per serving)

calories 15

fat 0 g 0%

protein 0 g 0%

carbohydrates 3.7 g 100%

fibers 0 g

Nachos sauce - Lactose free

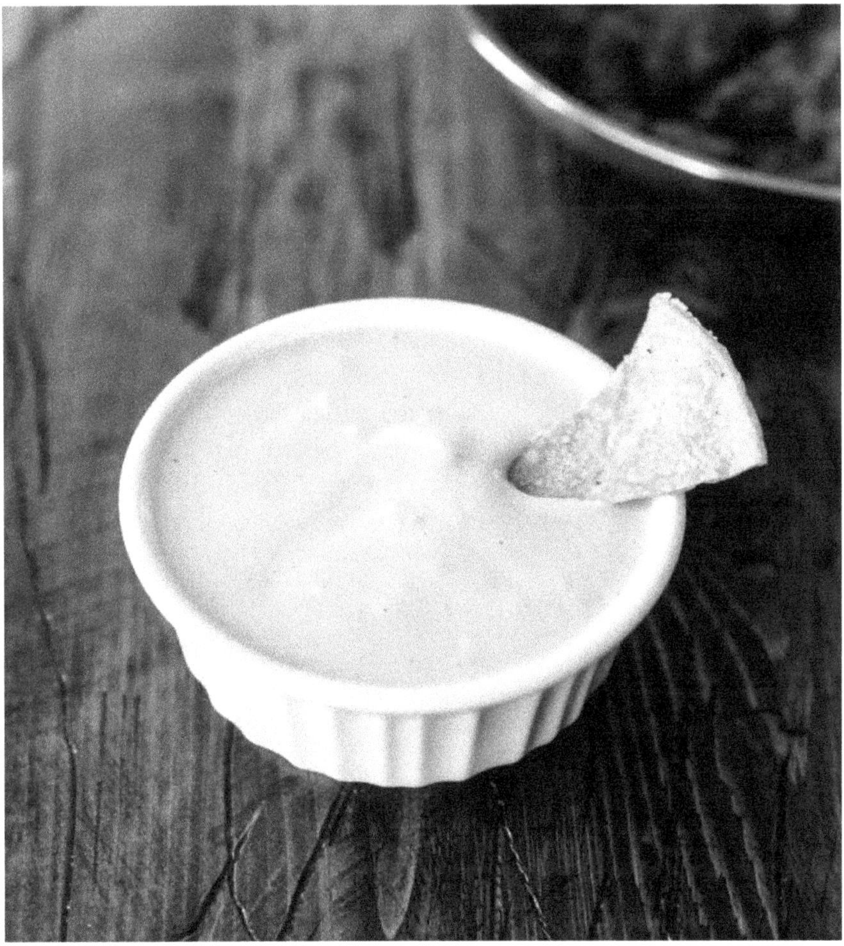

KETO - WITHOUT NUTS - WITHOUT LACTOSE

Preparation time: 2 minutes

Cooking time: 5 minutes

Yield: 2 cups (about ¼ cup per serving)

6 large egg yolks

¼ cup of lime or lemon juice

1 tablespoon of mustard

1 1/2 cups bacon or duck fat, melted (but not too hot)

¼ cup of nutritional yeast

½ teaspoon of fine sea salt

¼ teaspoon of taco seasoning

1. Making this cheese sauce is like making hollandaise sauce. At the bottom of a double boiler or in a medium-sized saucepan, bring 1 inch of water to a boil over high heat, then adjust the heat to keep it boiling. Place the egg yolks, lime juice, and mustard in the top of the double boiler or in a heat-resistant bowl that fits into the saucepan with the boiling water.

2. Beat the yolk mixture to blend, then, stirring constantly, add the melted fat in a slow, steady stream (this should take about 90 seconds). Cook the sauce, beating, until it reaches 60 ° C.

3. Add the nutritional yeast, salt and seasoning to the taco and continue whisking until thickened, about 3 minutes, adjusting the heat to maintain the temperature at 60 ° F (remove from boiling water if necessary) . Adjust the toppings to taste. Remove from heat and keep warm until ready to serve.

4. Store in an airtight container in the refrigerator for up to 2 weeks. Gently heat on the stove over low heat.

Nutritional information (per serving)

416 calories

fat 42.4 g 92%

proteins 4,7 g 5%

carbohydrates 3,9 g 4%

fibers 1.4 g

Baconnaise imitation

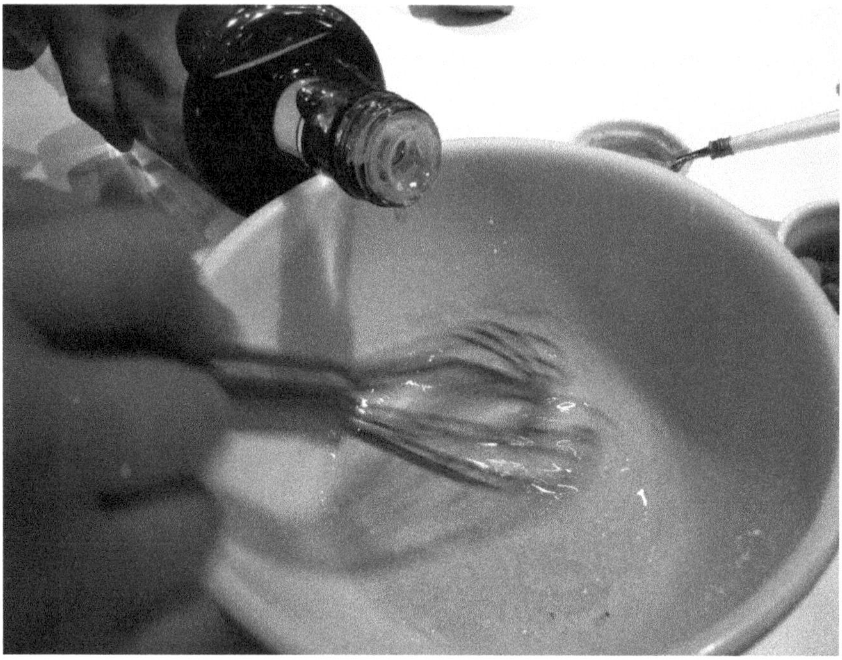

KETO - WITHOUT NUTS - WITHOUT LACTOSE

Preparation time: 5 minutes

Yield: 1¼ cups (1 tablespoon per serving)

2 large egg yolks

3 teaspoons of lemon juice, divided

1 cup bacon fat, melted (but not too hot)

Fine sea salt (if needed)

Necessary material

KITCHEN ROBOT

1. Place the egg yolks in a small food processor with 1 teaspoon of lemon juice and mix until well blended.

2. Turn on the food processor over low heat and slowly pour the melted bacon fat into the yolk mixture, drop by drop at the beginning. If you add too much oil at once, it will separate.

3. As you add more bacon fat, the mixture will begin to emulsify and thicken, so you can start pouring the fat in a steady stream.

4. After adding all the bacon fat, add the remaining 2 teaspoons of lemon juice. Taste and add salt as needed.

5. Store in the refrigerator and use within 5 days.

Nutritional information (per serving)

120 calories

fat 13.3 g 100%

protein 0 g 0%

carbohydrates 0 g 0%

fibers 0 g

Brown butter Bernese

KETO - WITHOUT NUTS

Preparation time: 5 minutes

Cooking time: 20 minutes

Yield: 3 cups (3 tablespoons per serving)

This recipe uses brown butter instead of regular butter for a richer flavor. I recommend keeping a jar of brown butter in the refrigerator for easy use in recipes. It's a great staple!

1 brown butter recipe

1/4 cup chopped fresh tarragon or sage

2 shallots, chopped

¼ cup of coconut vinegar or white wine vinegar

12 large egg yolks

Fine sea salt

Necessary material

MIXER

1. Place the brown butter in a medium-sized saucepan and melt it over medium heat. Add the tarragon, shallot and vinegar and bring to a boil. Cook for 15 minutes. Remove from heat and set aside to cool slightly.

2. Put the egg yolks in a blender. With the blender on medium speed, add a third of the brown butter mixture in a continuous stream. Once emulsified, increase the speed of the blender and add the remaining butter in a slightly faster stream. Season with salt to taste.

Tip: To make this sauce by hand, beat the egg yolks in a large bowl. Then, stirring vigorously, slowly add the brown butter reduction in a slow, steady stream. Once emulsified, you can pour the reduction faster. Season with salt to taste.

Variation: milk-free béarnaise. Instead of brown butter, use 1/2 cup of lard or bacon fat.

Nutritional information (per serving)

calories 93

fat 9.1 g 88%

protein 2.2 g 9%

carbohydrates 0.9 g 4%

fibers 0 g

Brown butter

KETO - WITHOUT NUTS

Cooking time: 5 minutes

Yield: ½ cup (2 tablespoons per serving)

In France, brown butter is called beurre noisette, which means "nut butter", referring to the brown color of hazelnut peels. It is simply butter that is heated until the milk proteins are golden brown and some of the water evaporates. It adds a rich nutty flavor to recipes that call for butter and can be used on its own as a hot sauce to accompany many foods, such as vegetables, fake pasta (such as zucchini "Pasta"), fish, omelettes and chicken. I also put a twist on homemade mustards to make them more quiet.

Put the butter in a saucepan and heat over high heat for about 5 minutes. The butter will begin to sizzle and foam. Look closely at the brown spots and once you see them, remove the pan from the heat and whisk vigorously. Be careful that the specks do not turn black: it means that it has started to burn and has turned into black butter or beurre noir (it's common in French cuisine, but to me it tastes like burnt). Add a pinch of salt to taste.

½ cup (1 stick) of unsalted butter

¼ teaspoon of fine sea salt

nutritional information (per serving)

208 calories

fats 23 g 99%

protein 0.3 g 1%

carbohydrates 0 g 0%

fibers 0 g

Chimichurri fat burning sauce

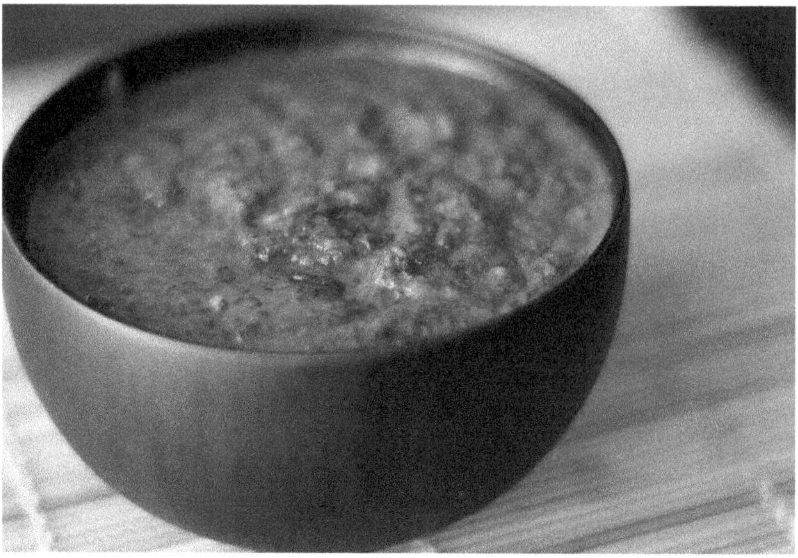

KETO - WITHOUT NUTS - WITHOUT LACTOSE

Preparation time: 5 minutes, plus 1 hour to set

Yield: 2 cups (about 2 tablespoons per serving)

Sauces and salad dressings are an easy and tasty way to turn a "low carb" meal into a "ketogenic" one by adding healthy and flavorful fats. A steak alone wouldn't have enough fat to make up a ketogenic dinner, but adding a flavorful, high-fat sauce turns it into a satisfying ketogenic meal. This Argentinian garlic-flavored sauce is great to serve not only with steaks but also with chicken, fish or seafood. It is also a great sauce for zucchini noodles.

1 roasted head of garlic or 3 raw garlic cloves, peeled

1 packed cup of fresh flat leaf parsley

½ cup of MCT oil

⅓ cup of coconut vinegar

¼ cup packed fresh cilantro

¾ teaspoon of red pepper flakes

½ teaspoon of ground cumin

½ teaspoon of fine sea salt

Necessary material

KITCHEN ROBOT

1. Squeeze the roasted garlic cloves from the head in a food processor (or put the raw garlic cloves in the food processor). Add the rest of the ingredients and whisk until smooth. Transfer to a serving bowl.

2. Cover and let sit at room temperature for up to an hour to allow the flavors to blend. Store in an airtight container in the refrigerator for up to 2 weeks.

Nutritional information (per serving)

calories 67

fat 7.1 g 95%

protein 0.2 g 1%

carbohydrates 0.5 g 39%

fibers 0 g

Enchilada sauce

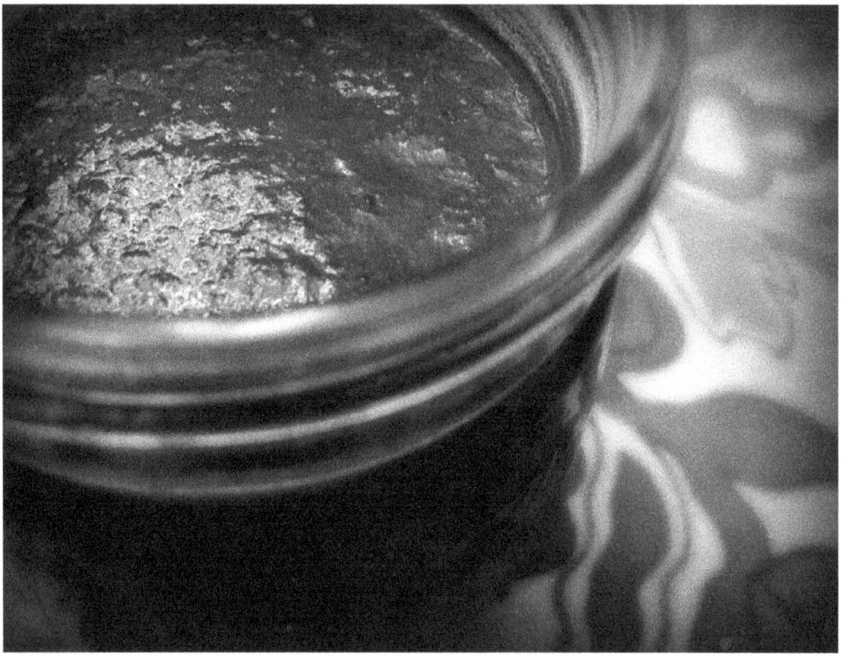

KETO - WITHOUT NUTS - WITHOUT LACTOSE

Preparation time: 10 minutes

Cooking time: 15 minutes

Yield: About 3 cups (1/4 cup per serving)

I have had many recipe testers who have tried multiple enchilada sauce recipes, and this one has been the winner over and over again! Using homemade bone broth is the key to creating a thick and flavorful sauce. Store-bought broth will work, but the end result won't be as thick. It is also important to check the ingredients in store-bought broths; many contain MSG and other harmful ingredients.

Put all the ingredients in a food processor and blend until smooth. Pour the sauce into a saucepan and heat slowly for about 15 minutes to thicken.

2 cups of chicken broth or beef bone broth

1 cup diced yellow tomatoes

½ cup chopped avocado (about ½ avocado)

1 head of roasted garlic

5 tablespoons of chili powder

2 tablespoons of fresh oregano or ½ teaspoon dried

2 tablespoons of lard, duck fat or other melted fat

1 tablespoon of coconut vinegar

½ teaspoon of ground cumin

Necessary material

KITCHEN ROBOT

Busy Families Tip: This recipe doubles up well, so make an extra for leftovers or freeze in pint jars.

Nutritional information (per serving)

calories 59

fats 4,2 g 64%

proteins 1,6 g 11%

carbohydrates 3.7 g 25%

fibers 2 g

Seasoning for taco

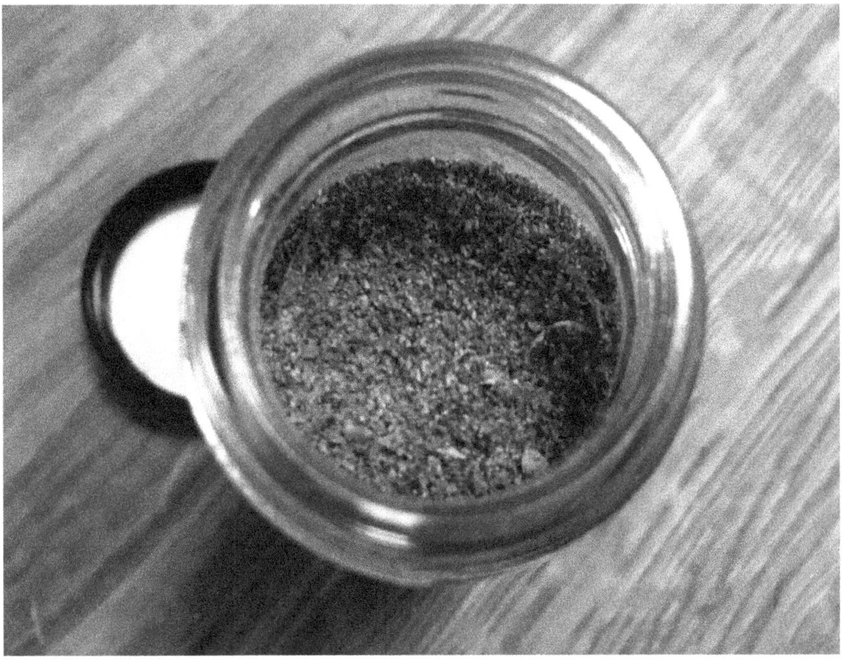

KETO - WITHOUT NUTS - WITHOUT LACTOSE

Preparation time: 2 minutes

Yield: ½ cup (1 tablespoon per serving)

When I use spice blends, I expect them to be made from spices. Doesn't seem to ask too much, does it?

See the following list of ingredients in store-bought taco seasoning: yellow cornmeal, salt, maltodextrin, paprika, spices, modified corn starch, sugar, garlic powder, citric acid, autolyzed yeast extract, natural flavor, color caramel (sulphites).

They don't even list a spice down to the fourth ingredient! But there are other problems too. Firstly, caramel dye is a food dye that has been linked to an increased risk of cancer.

Another problem is maltodextrin. Sugar has a glycemic index of 52, while that of maltodextrin is 110!

I'll just make a triple batch of my taco dressing and keep it in my pantry.

In a bowl, mix all ingredients until well combined. Store in an airtight container away from sources of heat and light for up to 2 months.

2 tablespoons of chili powder

1 tablespoon of ground cumin

2 teaspoons of fine sea salt

2 teaspoons of freshly ground black pepper

1 teaspoon of paprika

1 tsp ground coriander

½ teaspoon of garlic powder

½ teaspoon of onion powder

½ teaspoon of red pepper flakes

½ teaspoon of dried ground oregano

2 tsp powdered erythritol (optional)

Nutritional information (per serving)

calories 16

fats 0,6 g 34%

proteins 0.5 g 12%

carbohydrates 2.2 g 55%

fibers 1.1 g

Sea dressing

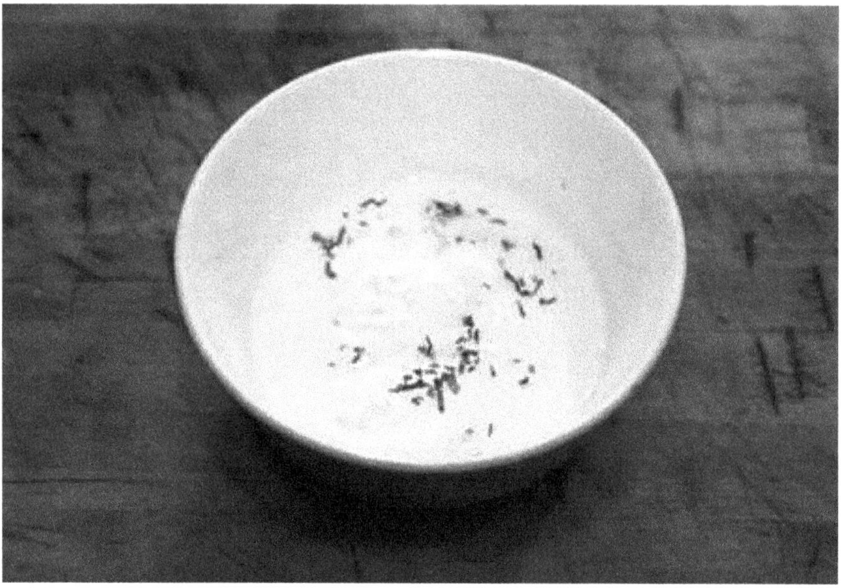

KETO - WITHOUT NUTS - WITHOUT LACTOSE

Preparation time: 2 minutes

Yield: 1 cup (1 tablespoon per serving)

Put all the ingredients in a bowl and mix well. Store in an airtight container, preferably away from sources of heat and light. It keeps for 3 months, but it is best to use it within 1 month.

¼ cup of smoked paprika

3 tablespoons of fine sea salt

3 tablespoons of garlic powder

2 tablespoons of onion powder

2 tablespoons of dried ground oregano

2 tablespoons of dried ground thyme

1 ½ tablespoon of freshly ground black pepper

1 1/2 tablespoons of cayenne pepper

Nutritional information (per serving)

calories 23

fats 0.4 g 16%

proteins 0,8 g 14%

carbohydrates 4 g 70%

fibers 1,5 g

How to store herbs

Freezing and drying herbs are great ways to store them for the long winter months. Drying works best for hard or "woody" herbs, which are suitable for long cooking times, although I have also found that they freeze well. Hard herbs include oregano, rosemary, sage, and thyme. Freezing is ideal for soft herbs, which are added towards the end of cooking or used raw on the finished dish. Soft herbs include basil, chives, dill, lovage, mint, parsley, and tarragon.

I often freeze all my herbs, but no matter what you do, I highly recommend skipping those expensive spice shops and going to the nearest farmers market to buy organic herbs. (Not all stalls at farmers' markets are organic; be sure to look for a sign or ask.) It's important to use organic herbs because, as with foods like lettuce, celery, and peppers, you eat the whole plant. It is less important to buy organic products when the food is protected by a thick, inedible outer skin, such as avocados or bananas.

The little time spent freezing and drying herbs is worth the money saved and the fresh taste in the dead of winter!

Dried herbs - freezing

STEP 1: Purchase or harvest organic herbs.

STEP 2: Rinse the herbs in water. Gently dry them or do what my mom does and gently dry them in a salad spinner (loves kitchen gadgets, while I'm minimalist). Be careful not to crush them.

STEP 3: Using your fingers, remove the leaves from the stems.

STEP 4: Place the leaves on a baking sheet rimmed in a single layer. Put in the freezer.

STEP 5: Once frozen, place the herbs in glass containers or jars, making sure to label and date them. (Freeze dried herbs often look alike.) Store in a dark pantry. For best flavor, use within 6 months.

Freezing herbs in oil

STEPS 1–3: Follow steps 1 to 3 for freeze drying herbs.

STEP 4: Place a tablespoon of leaves in each compartment of an ice cube tray, then fill each compartment with a tablespoon of high quality MCT oil or olive oil. Place the pan in the freezer.

STEP 5: Once frozen, place the herb-filled ice cubes in a glass container or one-gallon freezer bag, making sure to label and date it. Store in the freezer for up to 6 months.

Air drying herbs

STEPS 1–2: Follow steps 1 and 2 for freeze drying herbs.

STEP 3: Divide the herbs into small bunches, tying the ends with string.

STEP 4: Hang the bunches upside down in a clean area where they will not pulverize. If you're worried about dust, punch a hole in the bottom of a small paper bag and thread the string through the hole, leaving the top of the bag (now the bottom) open for air to circulate. Hang for several days until it dries; the exact time will vary depending on the temperature and humidity of the room they are hung in.

STEP 5: When the herbs are completely dry, munch the leaves off the stems.

STEP 6: Place the leaves in airtight glass containers, making sure to label and date them. For best flavor, use dried herbs within 6 months.

Tips

For a fresh taste of summer in the middle of winter, use frozen basil in olive oil cubes to make pesto and serve over the zucchini noodles.

When replacing dried herbs with fresh ones, use two-thirds less than the recipe requires. For example, if a recipe calls for 1 tablespoon of fresh thyme leaves, use 1 teaspoon dried.

Brown butter syrup

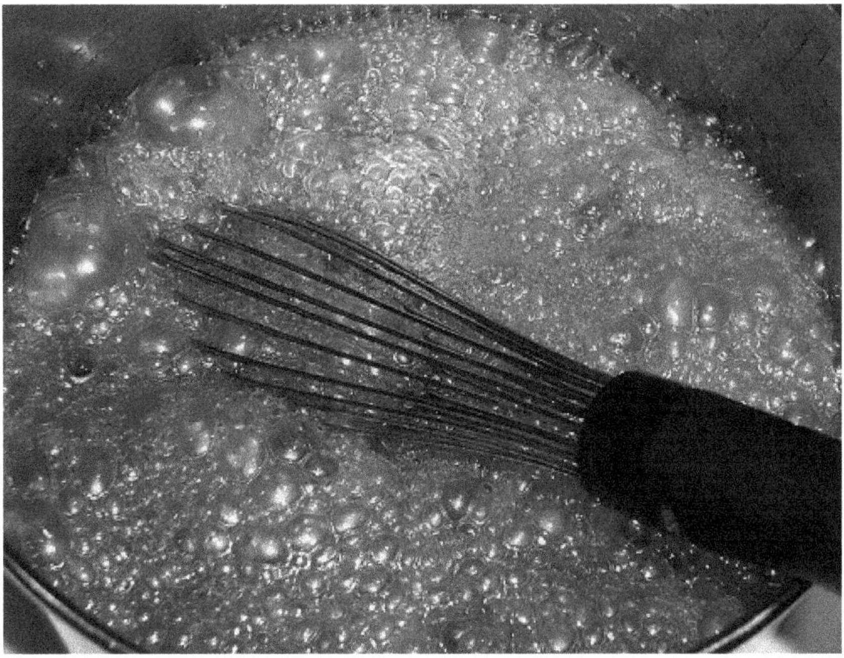

KETO

Preparation time: 1 minute

Cooking time: 5 minutes

Yield: 1 1/2 cups (2 tablespoons per serving)

To make brown butter syrup, I highly recommend using pastry-style sweetener. You can use pure erythritol, but when the syrup cools in the refrigerator, the almond milk will separate from the butter, which will solidify into pieces. If you decide to use a different sweetener, add half a kg of cream cheese to help the sauce emulsify.

½ cup (1 stick) of unsalted butter

½ cup of powdered erythritol

½ kg (2 tablespoons) of cream cheese (optional)

½ cup of unsweetened almond milk

1 teaspoon of maple extract or 2 drops of maple oil (optional)

¼ teaspoon of fine sea salt

1. In a large saucepan, heat the butter over high heat, whisking every few seconds. The butter will foam to the top of the saucepan and then fall back. When you see a lot of brown spots, remove from heat. Look carefully; you don't want black spots.

2. With the saucepan off the heat, beat the erythritol until smooth. If you used a brand of erythritol other than the pastry-style sweetener, add the cream cheese. Then add the almond milk, maple extract, if used, and salt.

3. Store in a glass jar in the refrigerator for up to 2 weeks if it lasts that long! This syrup will thicken in the refrigerator because the butter hardens as it cools; heat in a pan on the hob or in the microwave.

Nutritional information (per serving)

calories 77

fat 8,4 g 98%

protein 0.2 g 1%

carbohydrates 0.2 g 1%

fibers 0 g

CPSIA information can be obtained
at www.ICGtesting.com
Printed in the USA
BVHW060315020321
601390BV00006B/83

9 781802 113600